KATE HACKS:
- These procedures, whether you like it or not, are your new best friends as an aide, so you need to make sure that you study accordingly.
- I made flashcards and a **Quizlet** for all the little steps found in the RCPs that may be missed. You can find this at **quizlet.com** with the title **RCP Review Specifics** and the account **katesets**. This may be helpful if you don't want to make your own or need a different study tool. It is also a good thing to have when you just can't get yourself to study a whole RCP.
- Have your family and friends quiz you as much as possible. Even if you have 5 minutes of free time, use it to study. The repetition will help you to remember the many steps found in the RCP's.
- If you do not have anyone to quiz you, there is always studying by imagery and imagining yourself in the room you will be testing in. Picturing yourself doing an activity is creating a muscle memory as if you are actually doing the procedure.
- Focus on the skills that you don't want to study. A skill such as bed bath may look intimidating, but if you force yourself to study then on test day when you pull that skill, you will be well prepared.
- In my review classes, we play a "game" with the RCPs that I will share with you:
    - Write down an RCP on a piece of paper and place them all in a basket.
    - Randomly pick a piece of paper out and write down that RCP from memory.
    - You can then check what you got wrong and write those missed or incorrect steps in another color to visually see your mistake.
    - This will give you another way to study and a different way to see these skills.
- This is important:
    -

- The tester will test you on **WHAT YOU DO versus WHAT YOU SAY.**
- For example, if you go to put the gown on the residents affected left arm first but you say "I am putting the gown on the unaffected arm first" you will not be stopped because you are **DOING IT RIGHT** even though you are saying it wrong!

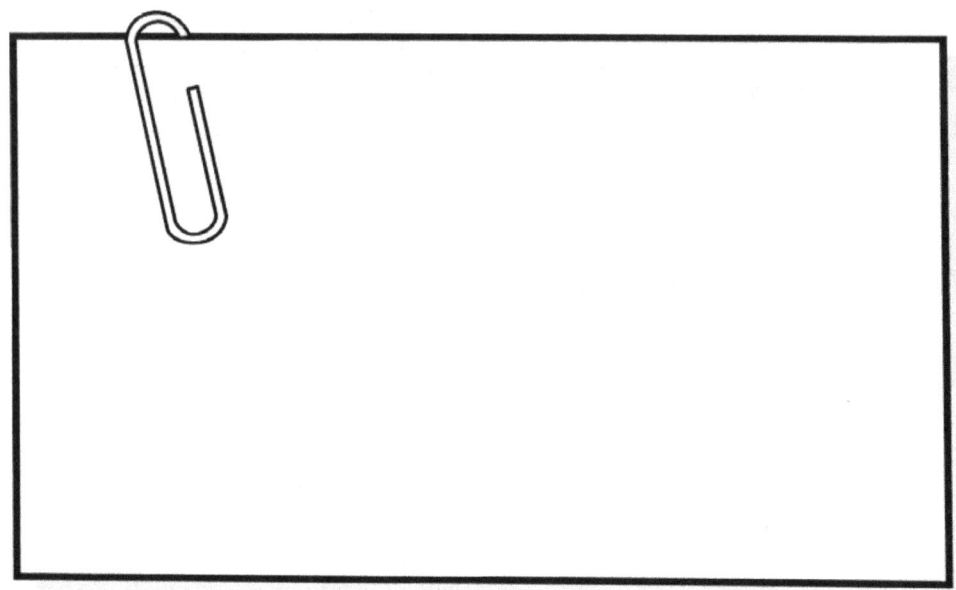

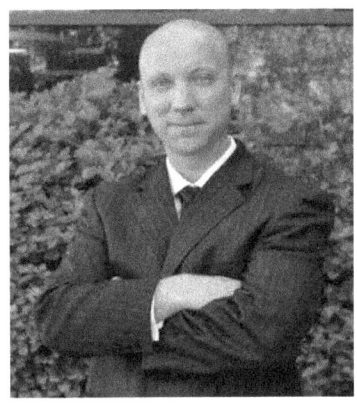

Chris Palevich, MBA, MSM
Executive Director
Premier Nursing Academy

FOREWORD:
Premier Nursing Academy emerged from the onslaught of the U.S. Department of Education and Obama Administration's rules aimed at reining in for-profit colleges. Although, this current administration might have a different agenda, no one can deny we are over 1 trillion dollars in student loan debt and it's escalating each year! Most importantly, these schools which were scuttled severed a demographic that does not have the luxury of attending 4 year/traditional university. These students have been pushed aside and the entire Long-Term Care industry has been left scrambling as to where to find their entry level Nurses. Until now…

With the closure of Medtech College, a few of us went in our own direction. Premier Nursing Academy was initially financed by Robert Palevich who is the Chairman of the Board and my father. We dreamed of creating a new educational vertical; funded by the Long-Term Care industry. By doing so, we could build a post-secondary college with zero student debt. Premier trains for what's being hired for, nothing else. We train for our institutions needs, to fulfill their patient to staff ratios and provide them with the candidates that have a desire to learn.

Far too long, has the Certified Nurse's Aide been an ending point for so many. There is an Indiana State Statute, which requires any new CNA to have their class reimbursed by their first employer. Knowing this, we designed our classes, giving each facility the opportunity to pick and choose who they want, prior to enrollment in our classes. We then can guarantee, through a Promissory Note, a 6-month work commitment for their tuition being sponsored. Our goal was to transform the Nursing community from the ground up, by bringing in a more vibrant candidate who is already Nursing career bound. We believed if we could transition a Freshman Pre-Nursing student into a CNA role, we could not only give that candidate a free education, but provide all our partnered facilities with a superior employee for 4 years. Therefore, drastically reducing turnover, enhancing overall patient care and providing our student 4 years relevant work experience, prior to graduation.

To create such an institution, Juli Murphy, BSN, RN was a co-worker at Medtech College and was brought on first to roll out our Certified Nurse Aide program. With any business, we learned quite quickly about growing pains and how our instructors are the lifeline for proper education and superior pass rates. Through 6 months of trial and error we have been able to build a team which could challenge any reputable school in the State of Indiana. Later this year, we will be expanding our program offerings.

To build a different demographic we needed to look at soon-to-be high school graduates who were entering the Nursing industry to expand our student base. In doing so, Katlyn Setser enrolled in our 3rd class and outshined all her peers. After finishing her written and skills tests flawlessly, she was hired as our Peer RCP reviewer. Katlyn has been able to maintain a 100% pass rate for anyone taking her courses, prior to testing.

Through Juli Murphy BSN, RN and Katlyn Setser's CNA leadership, we have been able to have a substantial impact in creating and maintaining new CNA applicants throughout Northeastern Indiana. Utilizing the Instructor's (Juli) feedback with how the student (Katlyn) learns philosophy; we have been able to develop an unparalleled teaching technique, with verifiable results.

If this book finds you, we wish you the best on your new CNA career! We look forward to being able to serve you; enhancing your overall CNA applicant base soon!

Best Regards,

Chris Palevich, MBA, MSM
Executive Director
Premier Nursing Academy
CPalevich@PremierNursing.org

HOW TO USE THIS HACKS GUIDE

- This guide contains 46 of the 72 RCP's required by the State of Indiana that are the most commonly tested procedures pulled during our program testing.
- This guide is not meant to replace the _Indiana State Department of Health Nurse Aide Curriculum_ (2014). It is however meant to help the student learn what **NOT TO DO** during the skills exam, therefore learning what **TO DO RIGHT!**
- Initial/final steps and some steps that require hand washing have been removed.
    - Reasoning:
        - **Hand Washing** – completed 1 time at the beginning of the test. You may need to verbalize at appropriate times during testing
        - **Initial Steps** – completed prior to your 4 procedures at the beginning of the testing (1 time only)
        - **Final Steps** – completed after your 4 procedures have been successfully performed at the end of the testing (1 time only)
- **Test Hacks** - Hacks and hints by a Program Director/Instructor after months of collecting errors and missed steps seen during testing to benefit students utilizing and studying this guide.
- **Study Hacks** - Hacks and hints by a CNA/RCP Peer Reviewer after months of collecting errors and missed steps seen during RCP Reviews and peer to peer mentoring to benefit students utilizing and studying this guide.
- **Critical Missed Steps** - Important steps highlighted in red that students have consistently missed during testing.
- The "Glove" - this icon lets you know this is a procedure that requires gloves.

TEST DAY HACKS

- You will take your written exam first (90 minutes to complete)
- After you have completed your written exam you will go to an assigned conference/waiting room
- Please DO NOT LEAVE THE BUILDING or your exam will be terminated
- The tester will come to the conference/waiting room for any questions and answers
- For each procedure (4 total) and hand washing you may have
    - 2 stops and 2 cues **free and clear**
    - On the third stop your test is **terminated**
- You will find out your written exam score after you complete your skills test
    - You will not get a percentage grade
    - You will only know what areas were above or below 80% of passing
- Please be quiet and respectful while in the conference/waiting room area during the skills exam
- Please be **professional and supportive** of those students who pass and especially of those who do not pass!
- Please maintain a **positive and professional attitude** at all times!
- You may leave the building after you have completed the skills exam and have signed off on all documents requested by the tester

PROCEDURE #1: INITIAL STEPS

1. Ask nurse about resident's needs, abilities and limitations, if necessary and gather
necessary supplies.

During the test do not gather the supplies until you have finished the initial steps

2. Knock and identify yourself before entering the resident's room. Wait for permission to enter the resident's room.

3. Greet resident by name per resident preference.

The name of the resident during the test is ALWAYS Mr. or Mrs. Smith. Remember to ALWAYS use the name given by the tester.

4. Identify yourself by name and title.

Yes, you need to do this twice, but it is important because it allows the resident to know who is entering the room and also gives a formal greeting once you are face to face.

Do not say "Patient Care". State your given name as stated in the RCP. NEVER SAY "at our facility we do this or that", the tester is testing you on the RCP procedure only!

5. Explain what you will be doing; encourage resident to help as able.

6. Gather supplies and check equipment.

During the test perform step #7 first. Then gather your supplies for procedure #1.

7. Close curtains, drapes and doors. Keep resident covered, expose only area of resident's body necessary to complete procedure.

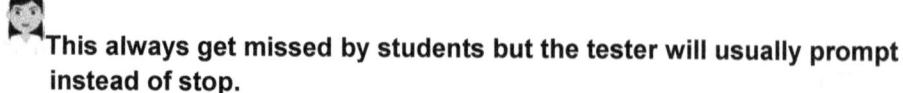This always get missed by students but the tester will usually prompt instead of stop.

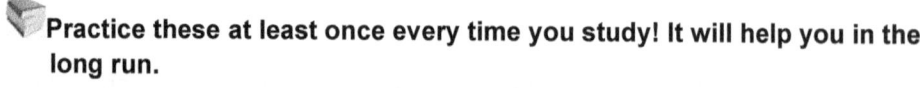Practice these at least once every time you study! It will help you in the long run.

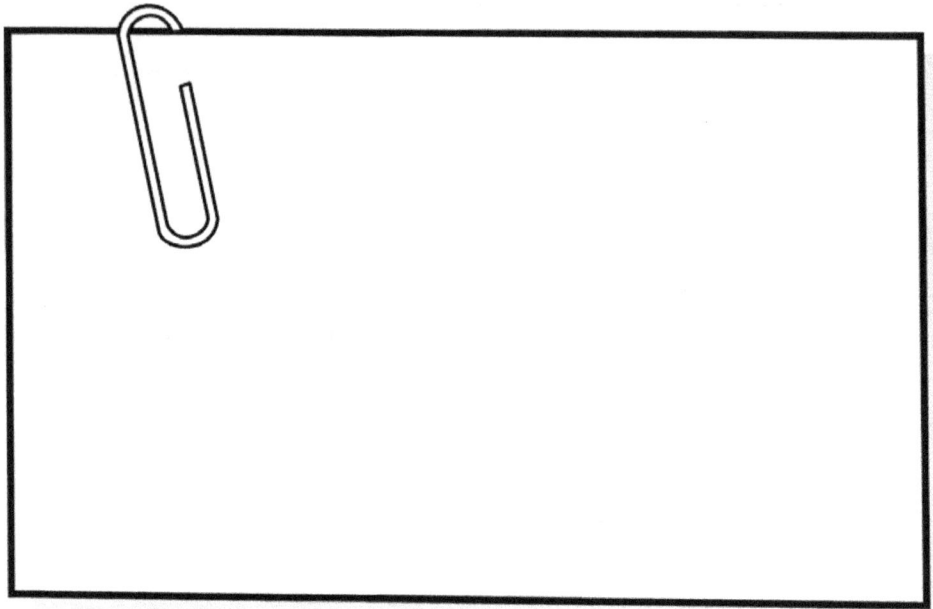

PROCEDURE #2: FINAL STEPS

1. Remove gloves, if applicable, and wash your hands.

2. Be certain resident is comfortable and in good body alignment. Use proper body mechanics

3. Lower bed height and position side rails (if used) as appropriate.

REMEMBER FOR ALL PROCEDURES: The resident is always safe when the bed is in the lowest position. Side rails do not need to be up during a test unless you are turning a resident.

4. Place call light and water within resident's reach.

5. Ask resident if anything else is needed.

6. Thank resident.

Believe it or not...this one gets missed a lot!

7. Remove supplies and clean equipment according to facility procedure.

8. Open curtains, drapes and door according to resident's wishes.

9. Perform a visual safety check of resident and environment.

Students will verbalize visual check but leave out the reason why... SAFETY!

10. Report unexpected findings to nurse.

11. Document procedures according to facility procedure.

Students are so excited that the skills exam is almost over they sometimes forget steps 10 and 11.

Practice these at least once every time you study! It will help you in the long run.

PROCEDURE #3: HANDWASHING

How to Hand wash (Wash hands when visibly soiled or prior to giving care)

1. Turn on faucet with a clean paper towel.

👩 Yes...you can use 1 paper towel to turn on both hot and cold faucets. **This gets asked a lot.**

2. Adjust water to acceptable temperature.

3. Angle arms down holding hands lower than elbows. Wet hands and wrists.

4. Apply enough soap to cover all hand and wrist surfaces. Work up a lather

NOTE: Direct caregivers must rub hands together vigorously, as follows, for at least 20 seconds, covering all surfaces of the hands and fingers.

👩 **The entire hand washing procedure should take 40 seconds. The scrub should take 20 seconds.**

♥ **5. Rub hands palm to palm.**

♥ **6. Right palm over top of left hand with interlaced fingers and vice versa.**

♥ **7. Palm to palm with fingers interlaced.**

♥ **8. Backs of fingers to opposing palms with fingers interlocked.**

♥ **9. Rotational rubbing, of left thumb clasped in right palm and vice versa.**

♥ **10. Rotational rubbing, backwards and forwards with clasped fingers of right hand in left palm and vice versa. Clean fingernails**

👩 **There are many steps to hand washing. Make sure you are performing all of them in front of the tester.**

11. Rinse hands with water down from wrists to fingertips

12. Dry thoroughly with single use towels.

♥ 13. Use towel to turn off faucet and discard towel.

Make sure you are not tempted to dry off your hands again after turning off the faucet with the paper towel (cross-contamination).

You can prevent this by putting your non-dominate hand behind your back while turning off the faucet and throwing the paper towel away.

Also, this can help because you do not want to touch the paper towel after you're done turning off the faucet...the tester can dock you for this!

Find your own order when practicing this procedure. If you practice in the same order every single time it will help with nervousness during the skills exam.

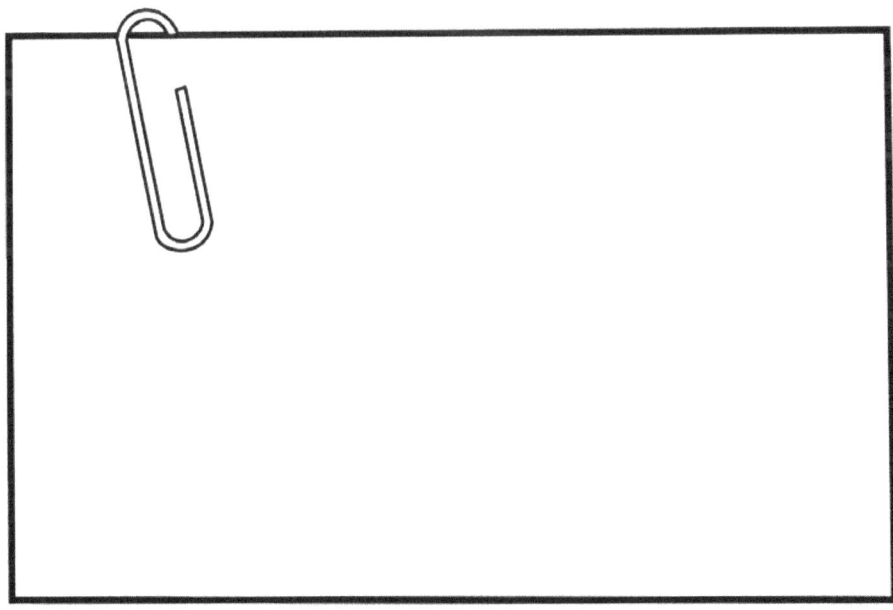

👋 PROCEDURE #4: GLOVES

2. If right-handed, slide one glove on left hand (reverse, if left-handed).

👩 Make sure the tester is watching you put on the gloves or you will have to repeat the procedure.

3. With gloved hand, slide opposite hand in the second glove.

♥ 4. Interlace fingers to secure gloves for a comfortable fit.

♥ 5. Check for tears/holes and replace glove, if necessary.

👩 If you fail to do steps 4 and 5 the tester will ask "is there something you would do for yourself for safety?".

6. If wearing a gown, pull the cuff of the gloves over the sleeves of the gown.

7. Perform procedure.

8. Remove first glove by grasping outer surface of the other glove, just below cuff and pulling down.

👩 Make sure you are just below the cuff when pulling off the glove, not at the palm or any other area of the glove...especially close to the skin!

9. Pull glove off so that it is inside out.

10. Hold the removed glove in a ball of the palm of your gloved hand. Do not dangle the glove downward.

11. Place two fingers of ungloved hand under cuff of the other glove and pull down, so, first glove is inside second glove.

👩 When putting 2 fingers under the cuff make sure they are pointing down along the palm of your hand, this way you will have less of a chance for the thumb to become contaminated by the dirty glove on the other hand... this has happened many times!

12. Dispose of gloves without touching outside of gloves and contaminating hands.

Make sure the tester watches you take off the gloves or you will have to repeat the procedure.

13. Wash hands.

The tester will say "what would you do for yourself?", this step has been missed.

When studying your RCP's, it may be best that you note which ones you will need gloves as there are a handful. The more procedures you need gloves for, the higher the chance of you getting this for your skills exam. This is important to know, even if it may seem like an easier skill.

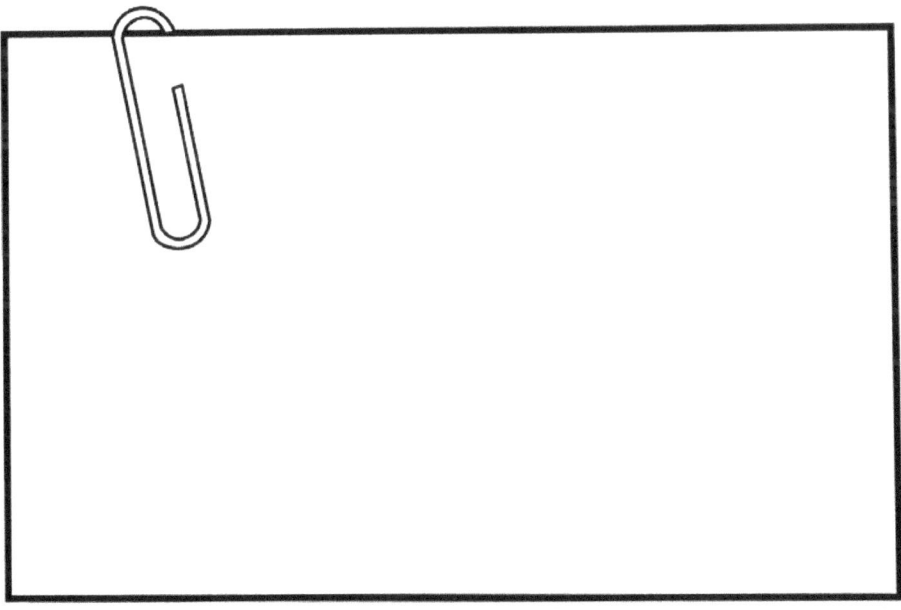

PROCEDURE #7: FALLING OR FAINTING

♥ 1. **Call for nurse and stay with resident.**

Many students want to check for breathing first and miss this step. ALWAYS call the nurse first!

Remember that all procedure skills require you to call for the nurse before you try and start anything else.

♥ 2. **Check if resident is breathing.**

This is the 2nd step...not the 1st. Many students check breathing first before calling for the nurse!

3. Do not move resident. Leave in same position until the nurse examines the resident.

4. Talk to resident in calm and supportive manner.

5. Apply direct pressure to any bleeding area with a clean piece of linen.

A lot of students during their review day tend to forget this simple task or place it before doing some of the others. Try and think about how you would really handle this situation. The order of these steps does make sense if you think about it.

♥ 6. **Take pulse and respiration.**

♥ 7. **Assist nurse as directed. Check resident frequently according to facility policy and procedures. Assist in documentation.**

It is the CNA's responsibility to take the pulse and respiration while the nurse is assessing the resident further.

PROCEDURE #8: CHOKING

♥ 1. Call for nurse and stay with resident.

📖 Remember that all procedure skills require you to call for the nurse before you try and start anything else.

👩 Students forget to call the nurse first!

♥ 2. Ask if resident can speak or cough.

👩 Asking if they can cough or talk will tell you if they can breathe. If they can cough or talk leave them alone to work it out on their own!

3. If not able to speak or cough, move behind resident and slide arms under resident's armpits.

4. Place your fist with thumb side against abdomen midway between waist and ribcage.

👩 For women this is right below the bra line.

5. Grasp your fist with your other hand.

♥ 6. Press your fist into abdomen with quick inward and upward thrust.

👩 Move in and up...NOT in and back!

7. Repeat until object is expelled.

👩 The tester will ask you "how long will you continue this?".

8. Assist with documentation.

PROCEDURE #9: SEIZURES

♥ 1. **Call for nurse and stay with resident.**

▸ Remember that all procedure skills require you to call for the nurse before you try and start anything else.

👩 Students forget to call the nurse first!

♥ 2. **Place padding under head** and move furniture away from resident.

♥ 3. Do not restrain resident or place anything in mouth, **assist nurse with placing resident on his/her side**

♥ 4. **Loosen resident's clothing especially around neck.**

♥ 5. **Note duration of seizure and areas involved.**

👩 Students forget what to do for residents during seizures (steps 2-5). If you think about the resident's safety and health it should come natural. Protect the head first, assist to their side so they won't choke on fluids, loosen clothing around the neck for airway!

PROCEDURE #10: FIRE

1. Remove residents from area of immediate danger.

2. Activate fire alarm.

3. Close doors and windows to contain fire.

4. Extinguish fire with fire extinguisher, if possible.

5. Follow all facility policies.

This sometimes get missed in the "RACE" acronym protocol.

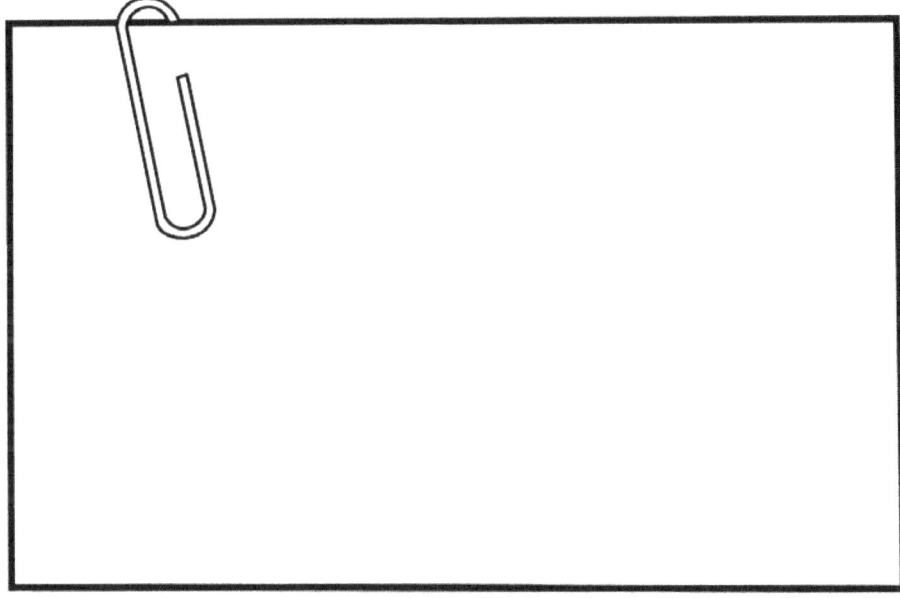

PROCEDURE #11: FIRE EXTINGUISHER

1. Pull the pin.

2. Aim at the base of the fire.

3. Squeeze the handle.

4. Sweep back and forth at the base of the fire.

Usually the "RACE" acronym is used and the tester will state "a fire has broken out what will you do?". However, you should always know the PASS acronym as well!

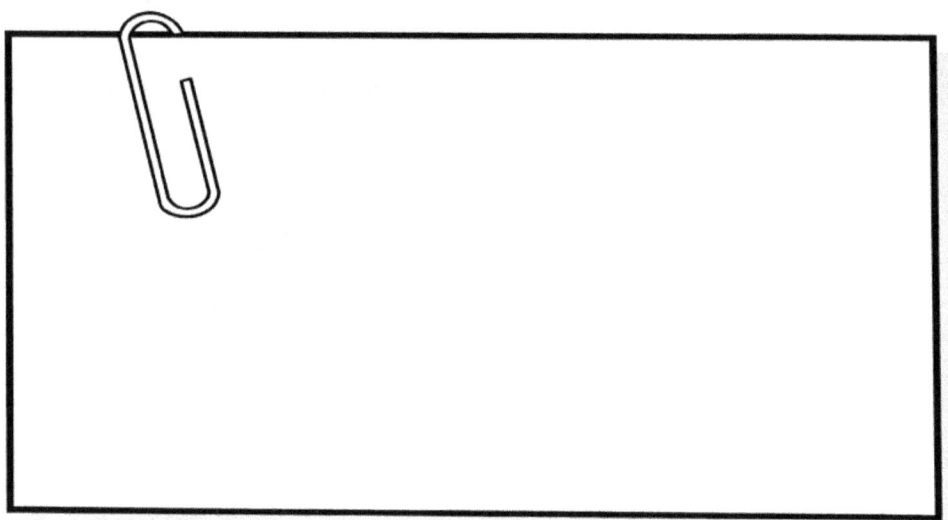

PROCEDURE #13: AXILLARY TEMPERATURE

1. Remove thermometer from storage/ battery charger.

3. Position resident comfortably in bed or chair.

4. Put on disposable sheath, remove resident's arm from sleeve of gown, wipe armpit and ensure it is dry. Hold thermometer in place with end in center of armpit and fold resident's arm over chest.

Make sure you remove the residents arm from the sleeve of the gown and bring a washcloth to wipe the arm pit.

Also, make sure you know how to put a disposable sheath on the thermometer and how to remove the outer paper to expose the plastic sheath.

5. Press button to activate the thermometer.

**You will actually be taking an axillary temperature during the test so PRESS
the button!**

6. Hold thermometer in place until signal is heard, indicating the temperature has been obtained.

7. Read the temperature reading on the face of the electronic device, remove the thermometer, discard the sheath, and record the reading.

Tell the tester your reading and he/she will have you document your finding on the testing procedure sheet. Know how to document a temperature!

8. Assist the resident to return arm through sleeve of clothing/gown.

10. Return thermometer to storage/battery charger.

11. Report unusual reading to nurse.

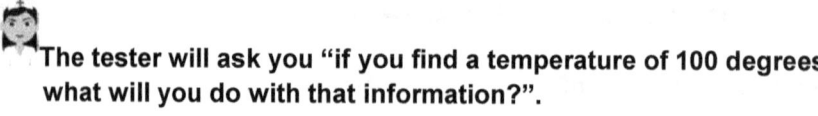The tester will ask you "if you find a temperature of 100 degrees what will you do with that information?".

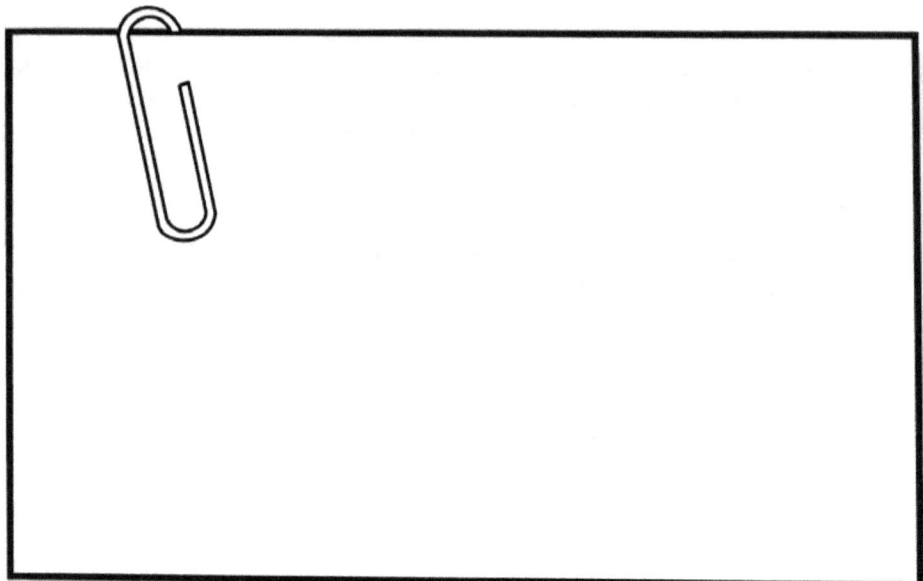

PROCEDURE #14: PULSE AND RESPIRATION

2. Place resident's hand on comfortable surface.

♥ 3. Feel for pulse above wrist on thumb side with tips of first three fingers.

Find the groove on the thumb side of the wrist using your index and middle fingers. Don't push too hard!

Have your watch with a second-hand ready.

When you are sure you have the pulse, tell the tester and he/she will find a pulse on the other wrist.

Tell the tester you are ready to start.

Count 1 full minute and then continue for 1 full minute to count respirations without stopping between pulse and respirations.

♥ 4. Count beats for 60 seconds, **noting rate, rhythm and force.**

Documenting characteristics has been missed.

♥ 5. Continue position as if feeling for pulse. **Count each rise and fall of chest, as one respiration.**

Students have stopped after the pulse to give the tester a pulse rate. This is wrong! Continue 1 minute more to count respirations.

♥ 6. Count respirations for 60 seconds noting **rate, regularity and sound.**

Documenting characteristics has been missed.

7. Record pulse and respiration rates.

The tester will have you document your findings on the testing procedure sheet.

8. Report unusual findings to nurse.

Know what is an unusual finding and what to report to the nurse as the tester will ask you this question.

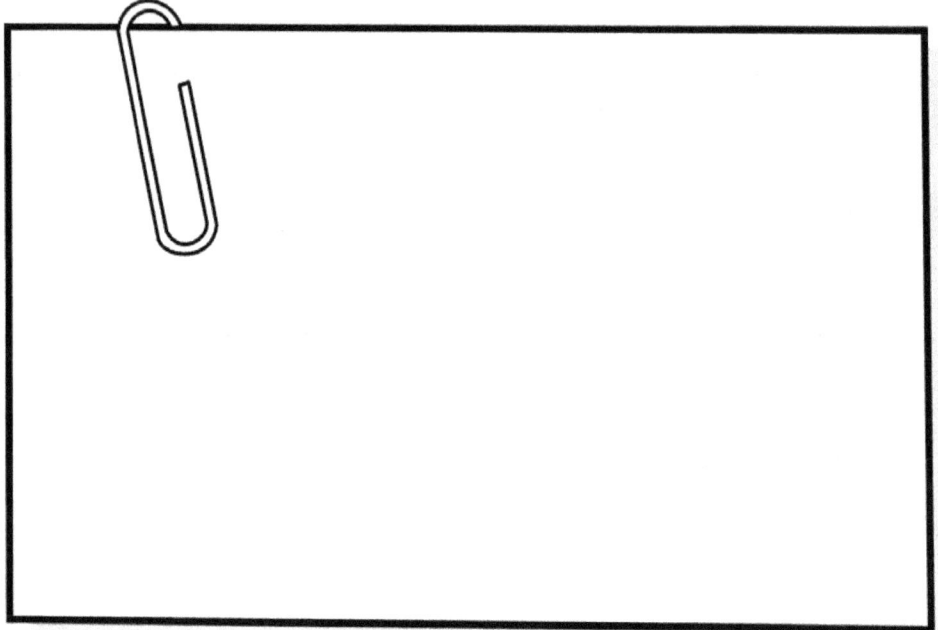

PROCEDURE #15: BLOOD PRESSURE

2. Clean earpieces and diaphragm of stethoscope with antiseptic wipe.

The teaching stethoscope is used because the tester will be listening with you...be prepared for this. Make sure you clean off the earpieces for the tester.

3. Uncover resident's arm to shoulder.

4. Rest resident's arm, level with heart, palm upward on comfortable surface.

5. Wrap proper sized sphygmomanometer cuff around upper unaffected arm approximately 1-2 inches above elbow.

Students have made many mistakes in this skill!
Be sure the cuff is 2" above the elbow, the arrow is pointing at the brachial artery, and be sure to have the cuff on tight enough. You WILL NOT get an accurate reading if this is not done correctly.

Practice your blood pressures till you can do them in your sleep!

6. Put earpieces of stethoscope in ears.

7. Place diaphragm of stethoscope over brachial artery at elbow.

Make sure you place the diaphragm over the bend/crease of the elbow. This is where you will hear the pulse best.

Make sure you hold the stethoscope firmly so you can hear the systolic and diastolic pressures. Practice holding your equipment at home so this does not feel clumsy to you.

There is an art to pumping the bulb, holding the stethoscope and reading the pressure all at once. You can do it but it takes practice! Once you have it... it's like riding a bicycle... you won't lose it!

8. Close valve on bulb. If blood pressure is known, inflate cuff to 20 mm/hg above the usual reading. If blood pressure is unknown, inflate cuff to 160 mm/hg.

Students have been stopped by the tester when pumping the cuff over 160mm/hg. **Make sure it is EXACTLY 160mm/hg!**

9. Slowly open valve on bulb.

A good tip for this is to close the valve as tight as it will go and then undo the valve just a small amount before beginning the blood pressure. This will help so that when taking the pressure, you will not let too much air out at once.

10. Watch gauge and listen for sound of pulse.

11. Note gauge reading at first pulse sound.

12. Note gauge reading when pulse sound disappears.

13. Completely deflate and remove cuff.

Make sure you deflate the cuff fully before finishing the procedure and verbalizing the blood pressure measurement.

14. Accurately record systolic and diastolic readings.

The tester will ask you to document your findings (example 120/80) on your testing procedure sheet.

16. Report unusual readings to nurse.

The tester will ask you "what would you do if the systolic pressure was over 200?"

PROCEDURE #17: WEIGHT

2. Balance scale.

Balance scale by ZERO-ing it out. If scale is digital you may step on it to apply enough pressure until ZERO appears.

3. Depending on scale used, assist resident to stand on platform or sit in chair with feet on footrest or transport wheelchair onto scale and lock brakes.

4. When using a standard scale –lower weight to fifty-pound mark that causes arm to drop. Move it back to previous mark. Move upper weight to pound mark that balances pointer in middle of square. Add lower and upper marks. When using a digital scale – press weight button. Wait until numbers remain constant.

5. Subtract weight of wheelchair from total weight, if applicable.

6. Accurately record resident's weight.

The tester will ask you to document your findings (example: 130.5 lbs.) on your procedure sheet.

8. Report unusual reading to nurse.

The tester will ask you "if the resident gained 5 pounds in 24 hours what would you do with that information?".

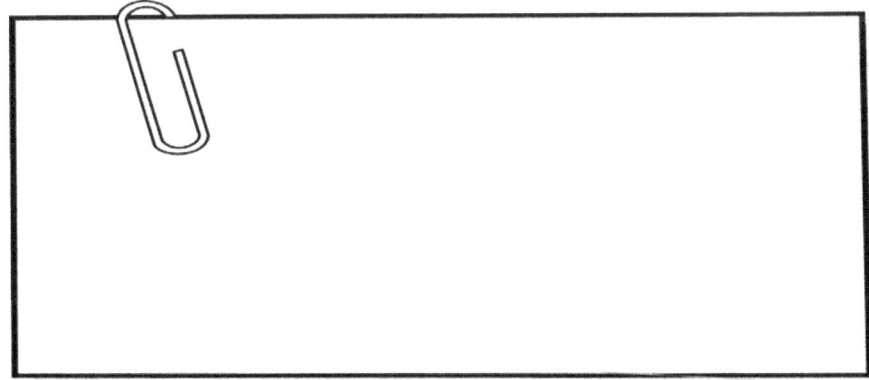

PROCEDURE #19: SUPINE POSITION

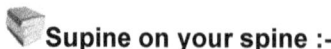 Supine on your spine :-)

2. Lower head of bed.

3. Move resident to head of bed if necessary.

♥ **4. Position resident flat on back with legs slightly apart.**

♥ **5. Align resident's shoulder and hips.**

Students have missed legs apart and aligned with shoulders and hips...this is a stop!

6. Use supportive padding and/or float heels, if necessary.

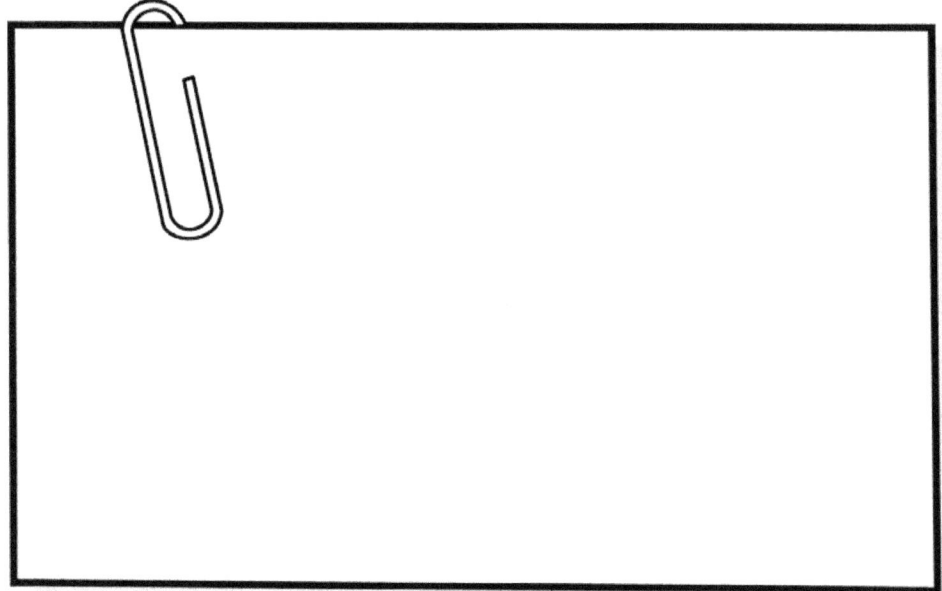

PROCEDURE #20: LATERAL POSITION

2. Place resident in supine position.

👧 **At this point, put the side rail up on the side you are going to turn the resident toward prior to turning them.**

👧 **Remember...you only put up the side rail during a test when you turn the resident!**

3. Move resident to side of bed closest to you.

4. Cross resident's arms over chest.

5. Slightly bend knee of nearest leg to you or cross nearest leg over farthest leg at ankle.

6. Place your hands under resident's shoulder blade and buttock. Turn resident away from you onto side.

👧 **No side rail would need to be up at this point as long as you are on the same side of the bed as a support/safety person.**

7. Place supportive padding behind back, between knees and ankles and under top arm.

👧 **Leave the side rail up on the residents anterior (forward facing) side for safety.**

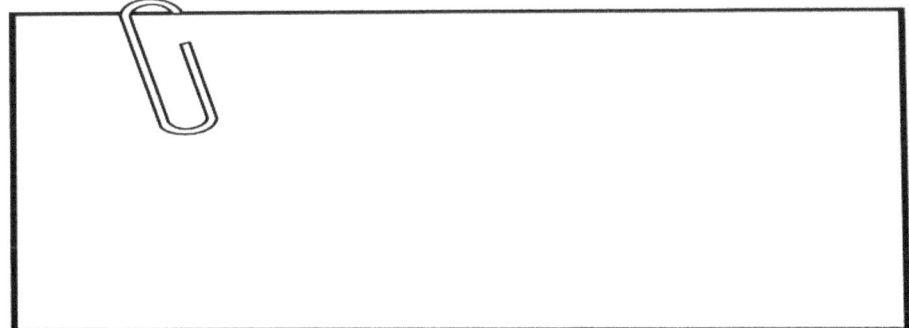

27

PROCEDURE #21: FOWLER'S POSITION

2. Move resident to supine position.

♥ 3. Elevate head of bed **45 to 60 degrees**.

📘 The degrees always go by 15.

👩 Use a magnetic gauge if available. The gauge should be placed on the movable bed part that you are moving. Verbalize to the tester that Fowlers is with the head of the bed elevated between 45-60 degrees. The tester will then check your positioning to make sure it is correct.

4. Use supportive padding if necessary.

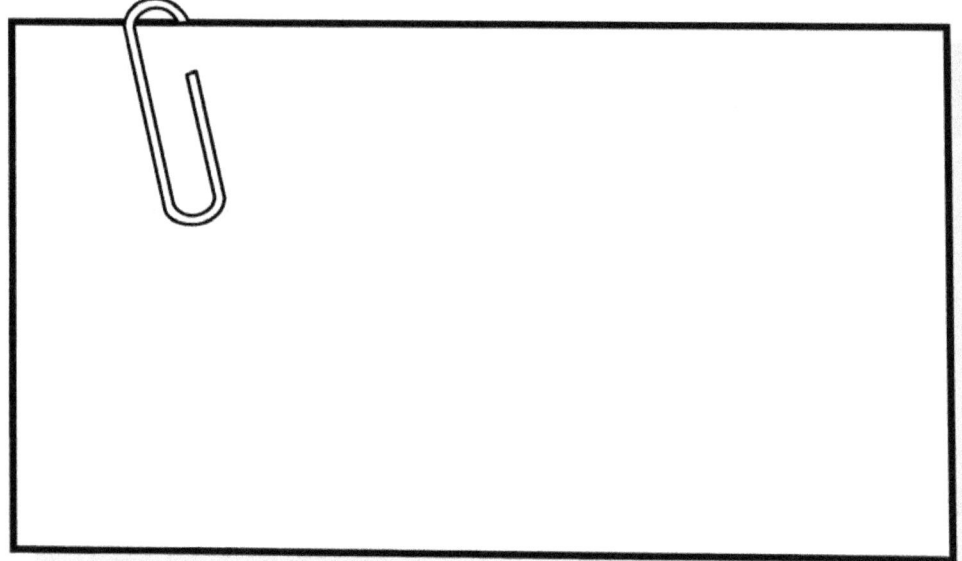

PROCEDURE #22: SEMI-FOWLER'S POSITION

2. Move resident to supine position.

3. Elevate head of bed **30 to 45 degrees**.

You can think of semi as only part of Fowlers. So, if you know that Fowlers is a larger degree just remember that semi-fowlers is just under that.

Use a magnetic gauge if available. The gauge should be placed on the movable bed part that you are moving. Verbalize to the tester that Semi-Fowlers is with the head of the bed elevated between 30-45 degrees. The tester will then check your positioning to make sure it is correct.

4. Use supportive padding if necessary.

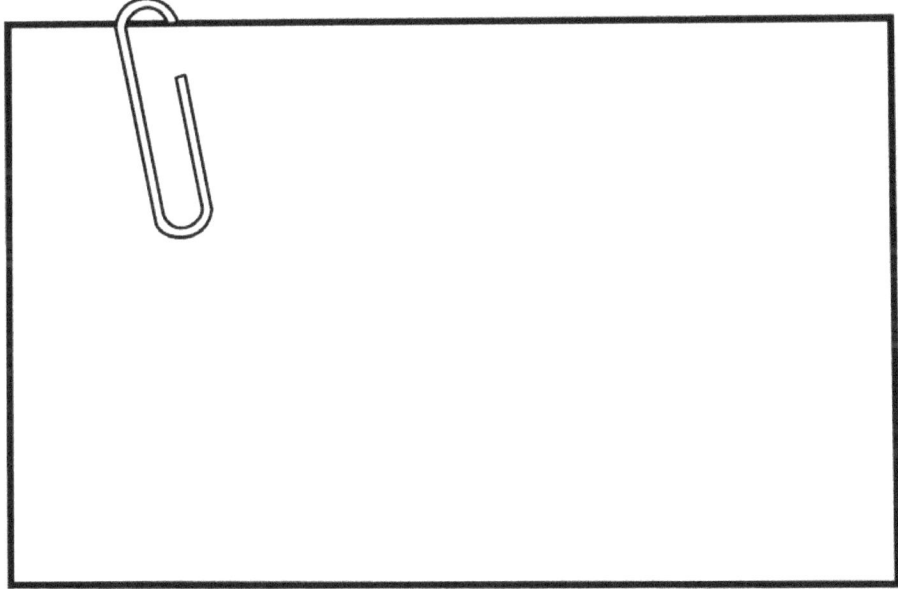

PROCEDURE #23: SIT ON EDGE OF BED

♥ 2. Adjust bed height to lowest position.

👩 This is the MOST TESTED procedure in the skills exam because it leads into other procedures.

👩 You should always leave bed in the lowest position/safest position during the test unless you are so tall that you must bend over at the waist or squat.

♥ 3. Move resident to side of bed closest to you.

👩 You may ask the resident to help you!

📖 Don't make this procedure harder on yourself. It is not easy to bring someone close to you in a bed.

♥ 4. Raise head of bed to sitting position, if necessary.

📖 If an RCP says, "if necessary" you should perform it on the skills exam. These are basically tips straight from State.

👩 Many students have forgotten to raise the head of the bed making this procedure very difficult.

♥ 5. Place one arm under resident's shoulder blades and the other arm under resident's thighs.

👩 Many students have missed hand placement on this! Stops have occurred when students have swung legs over and not placed their arm under both thighs.

♥ 6. On count of three, slowly turn resident into sitting position with legs dangling over side of bed.

Sitting up resident = counting to 3 ALWAYS!

7. Allow time for resident to become steady. Check for dizziness

When practicing this skill, you should practice asking if your resident is dizzy as well. Make it a habit to check for this, it is very important.

Always use the word dizzy i.e "Are you dizzy?"

Sitting up resident = checking for dizziness ALWAYS!

8. Assist resident to put on shoes or slippers.

Do not put shoes on while lying in bed (infection control stop). Always remember to put shoes on for stability after you sit them up at edge of bed with feet flat on floor.

9. Move resident to edge of bed so feet are flat on floor.

Make sure feet are flat on the ground and not dangling. This will not only help them, but it will make transferring easier on you.

PROCEDURE #24: USING A GAIT BELT TO ASSIST WITH AMBULATION

2. Assist resident to sit on edge of bed. Encourage resident to sit for a few seconds to become steady. Check for dizziness.

3. Place belt around resident's waist with the buckle in front (on top of resident's clothes) and adjust to a snug fit ensuring that you can get your hands under the belt. Position one hand on the belt at the resident's side and the other hand at the resident's back.

Students have let gait belt fall to floor while unwinding it (infection control stop).

Students have also put hands at both sides of resident while in front of resident and not one at their side and one at their back while standing to the side of resident.

4. Assist the resident to stand on count of three.

The resident needs to know what you are doing and when you are doing it. Counting gives them the timeframe to know when it is going to happen.

Standing a resident upright = counting to 3 ALWAYS!

5. Allow resident to gain balance. Ask the resident if dizzy.

Standing a resident upright = checking for dizziness ALWAYS!

6. Stand to side and slightly behind resident while continuing to hold onto belt.

Positioning is always important during the test. Standing to the side and slightly back is for safety in case the resident falls.

7. Walk at resident's pace.

8. Return resident to chair or bed and **remove belt**.

Students may be so excited the procedure is over they forget to remove the gait belt. The tester may prompt with "what does the resident no longer need?".

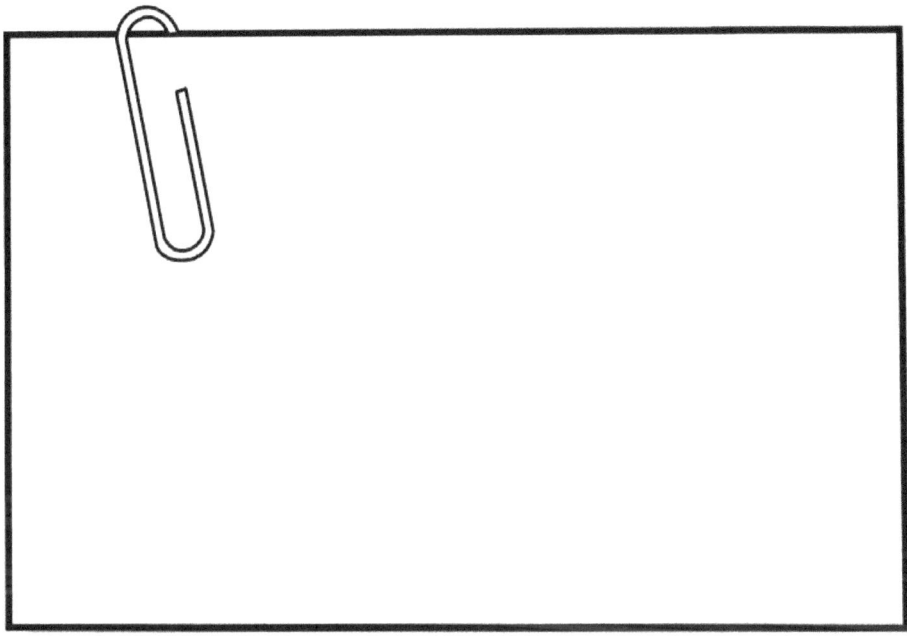

PROCEDURE #26: TRANSFER TO WHEELCHAIR

♥ **2. Place wheelchair on resident's unaffected side. Brace firmly against side of bed** with wheels locked and foot rests out of way.

Remember to always place a sitting device on the UNAFFECTED /STRONG side.

Students have failed this procedure with 1-2" left between the bed and wheelchair. MAKE SURE it is braced firmly with NO SPACE between the chair and bed.

Many times at a clinical site students may see facility CNA's transfer by placing the chair diagonally. This is wrong and unsafe. During testing it needs to be firmly against the bed. You can get a stop for this.

♥ **3. Assist resident to sit on edge of bed.** Encourage resident to sit for a few seconds to become steady. **Check for dizziness.**

Sitting a resident up = checking for dizziness ALWAYS!

Again, when studying for the exam be sure to practice asking if your resident is dizzy. It will become second nature to you when performing these skills.

♥ **4. Stand in front of resident and apply gait belt around the resident's abdomen**

Some students forget that this step DOES require a gait belt to transfer!

♥ **5. Grasp the gait belt securely on both sides of the resident**

I have seen some varied areas of grasping on the gait belt that have caused stops….remember you are standing in FRONT of the resident and you should grasp on both SIDES of the gait belt

♥ **6. Ask resident to place his hands on your upper arms.**

👩 Stops have occurred when students have failed to ask the resident to place their hands on the student's upper arm or have not suggested any placement at all.

♥ **7. On the count of three,** help resident into standing position by straightening your knees. **Stand toe to toe with resident**

👩 Standing a patient upright = counting to 3 ALWAYS!

👩 Students will forget foot placement on wheelchair...TOE TO TOE!

♥ **8.** Allow resident to gain balance, **check for dizziness.**

👩 Standing a resident in an upright position = checking for dizziness ALWAYS!

9. Move your feet to shoulder width apart and slowly turn resident.

10. Lower resident into wheelchair by bending your knees and leaning forward.

♥ **11. Align resident's body and position foot rests. Remove gait belt.**

👩 The tester may allow you to verbalize positioning of foot rest.

👩 Students are so excited the procedure is ALMOST over they forget to remove the gait belt. The tester may prompt "what is the resident no longer using?".

♥ **12.** Unlock wheels. **Transport resident forward through open doorway** after checking for traffic.

13. Transport resident up to closed door, open door and back wheelchair through doorway.

14. Take resident to destination and lock wheelchair.

Most of the time steps 12, 13 and 14 are verbalized to the tester. Please know them by memory. Students have had stops on these

Step 14 is not considered a restraint as you are locking the wheelchair once you reach the destination (ie: activity table) for safety.

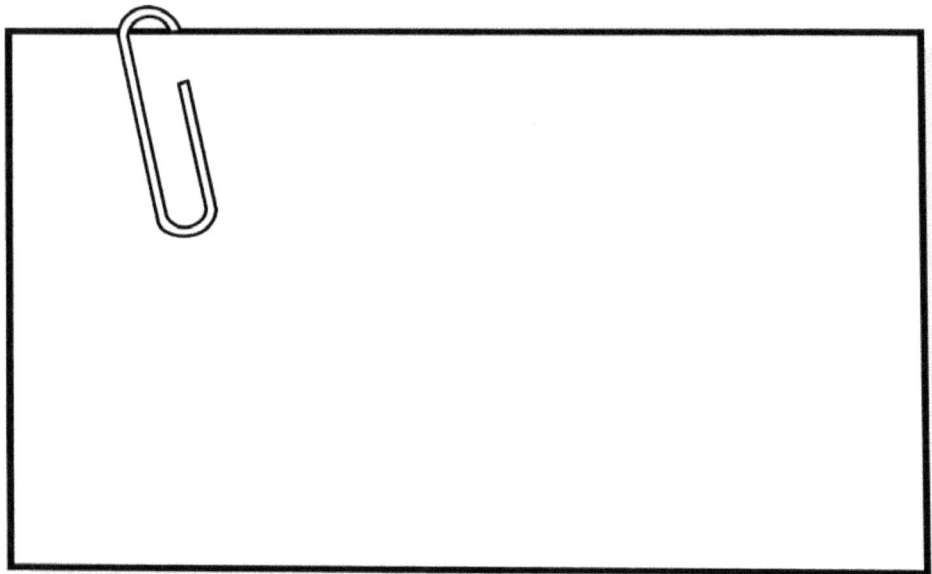

PROCEDURE #29: ASSIST WITH CANE

♥ 2. Check the cane for presence of rubber tip(s).

I have seen students stumble over this step. The tester will ask you "what would you check for prior to giving the resident a cane?"

3. Assist resident to sit on edge of bed.

♥ 4. Assist resident to stand on count of three.

Standing a resident to an upright position = counting to 3 ALWAYS!

♥ 5. Allow resident to gain balance. **Check for dizziness.**

Standing a resident to an upright position = checking for dizziness ALWAYS!

♥ 6. Have resident place cane approximately 4 inches to the side of his/her stronger/ unaffected foot. The height of the cane should be level with resident's hip.

During reviews students often ask why the cane is placed on the residents stronger side. If placed on their affected side they would not be able to properly support themselves with the cane.

♥ 7. Stand to the affected side and slightly behind resident.

You also stand on their affected side to help support them.

♥ 8. Have resident move cane forward about 4-6 inches, step forward with weak (affected) leg to a position even with the cane. Then have resident move strong leg forward and beyond the weak leg and cane. Repeat the sequence.

How far to have a resident move the cane is sometimes confused with a walker. A good rule to remember: a cane is > 6" and a walker is < 6".

Students also forget the process of which to move first... just remember you want to move the strong CANE first so it can support the affected/weak leg, then move the stronger leg through past the weak leg.

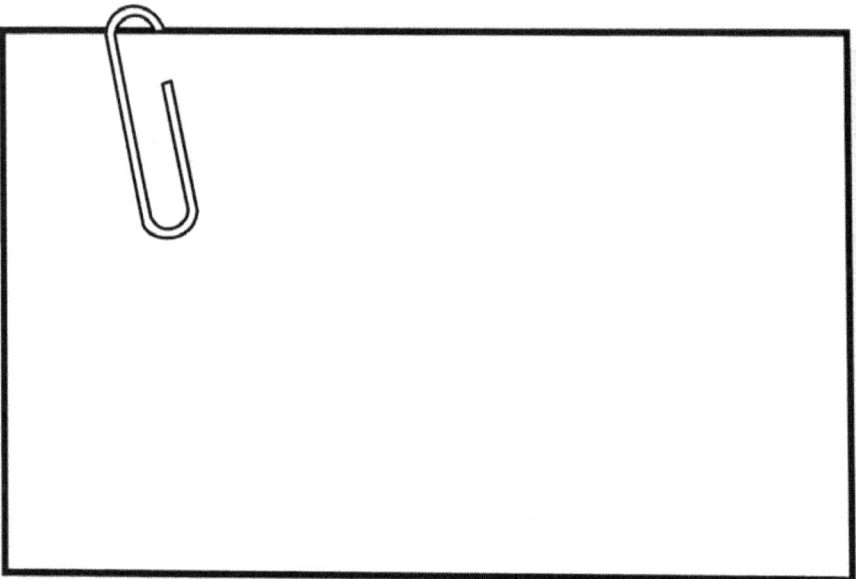

PROCEDURE #33: BED BATH/PERINEAL CARE

📖 This is one of those long RCPs that no one wants to study but you should. Writing down the body parts cleaned in order and when you change the water and gloves is a good way to study for this RCP.

♥ 2. Offer resident urinal or bedpan.

👧 This gets missed a lot. The resident may refuse this during the test, but you must remember to ask.

3. Provide Resident privacy

👧 Remember to pull down the sheet and blanket and utilize a bath blanket.

4. Fill bath basin with warm water and have resident check water temperature for comfort, if able.

📖 Always fill the bath basin halfway with water. The tester will ask you this.

5. Put on gloves.

📖 First set of gloves.

6. Fold washcloth and wet.

♥ 7. Gently wash eye from inner corner to outer corner, using a different part of cloth to wash the other eye.

👧 Many stops have occurred during this step from not using different parts of washcloth.

8. Wet washcloth and apply soap, if requested. Wash, rinse and pat dry face, neck, ears and behind ears.

👧 Remember to bring enough washcloths to change out for all areas of the body.

9. Remove resident's gown.

10. **Place towel under far arm.**

Many students have been stopped on this step. It is the only time you may reach across a resident that is not a safety caution stop.

11. Wash, rinse and pat dry hand, arm, shoulders and underarm.

Remember to wash up toward heart.

12. Repeat steps with the other arm.

13. Place towel over chest and abdomen. Lower bath blanket to waist.

Remember to bring enough bath and hand towels so you can place them under arms, legs, over chest etc. Privacy is very important! This cannot be stressed enough.

14. Lift towel and wash, rinse and pat dry chest and abdomen.

15. Pull up bath blanket and remove towel.

16. Uncover and place towel under far leg.

Make sure you are never exposing the resident. Always utilize the towels and bath blanket during the bath.

17. Wash, rinse and pat dry leg and foot. Be sure to wash, rinse and dry well between the toes.

18. Repeat with other leg and foot.

19. **Change bath water and gloves, wash hands and use clean gloves and towel.**

Do not forget this step prior to catheter care/perineal care

Second set of gloves

20. Assist resident to spread legs and lift knees, if possible.

21. Wet and soap folded washcloth.

Catheter Care:

22. If resident has catheter, check for leakage, secretions or irritation. Gently wipe four inches of catheter from meatus out.

Perineal Care:

23. Wipe from front to back and from center of perineum to thighs. If washcloth is visibly soiled, change cloths.

For Females:
- Separate labia. Wash urethral area first.
- Wash between and outside labia in downward strokes, alternating from side to side and moving outward to thighs. Use different part of washcloth for each stroke.

For Males:
A. Pull back foreskin if male is uncircumcised. Wash and rinse the tip of penis using circular motion beginning with urethra.
B. Continue washing down the penis to the scrotum and inner thighs. Rinse off soap and dry. Return foreskin over the tip of the penis.

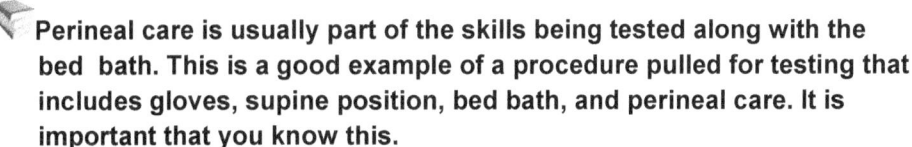Since the resident is usually a live person, the tester will ask you to verbalize these steps - know how to wash both male and female genitalia.

Perineal care is usually part of the skills being tested along with the bed bath. This is a good example of a procedure pulled for testing that includes gloves, supine position, bed bath, and perineal care. It is important that you know this.

24. Change water in basin. Wash hands and change gloves. With a clean

washcloth, rinse area thoroughly in the same direction as when washing.

📚 **Remember that when you fill a bath basin it is halfway.**

📚 **Third set of gloves**

25. Gently pat area dry with towel in same direction as when washing.

26. Assist resident to lateral position, facing away from you.

27. Wet and soap washcloth.

28. Clean anal area from front to back. Rinse and pat dry thoroughly.

29. Change bath water and gloves. Use clean washcloth and towel.

30. Wash, rinse and pat dry from neck to buttocks.

31. Return to supine position.

📚 **Supine on your spine :-)**

❤️ **32. Wash hands and change gloves**

📚 **Fourth glove change**

👩 **Note how many times you change gloves - 4 total.**

👩 **Bring 4 sets of gloves with you when you gather supplies.**

33. Help resident put on clean gown.

35. Report any reddened areas, abrasions or bruises to the nurse.

👩 **This procedure does not get pulled a lot but when it does it seems overwhelming to the student. Take a deep breath and make sure you MEMORIZE all steps!**

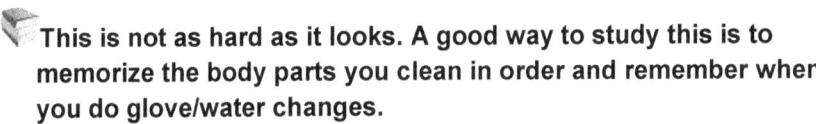 This is not as hard as it looks. A good way to study this is to memorize the body parts you clean in order and remember when you do glove/water changes.

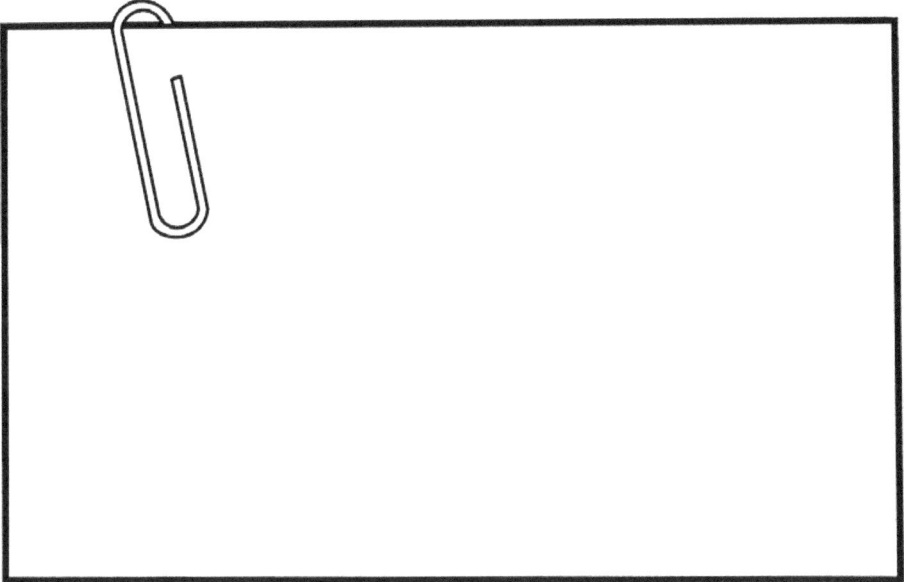

PROCEDURE #34: BACK RUB

♥ 2. Place resident in lateral position with neck/back toward you.

👩 Put your side rail up before turning resident

3. Expose back and shoulders.

4. Rub lotion between your hands.

📖 You are doing this to warm the lotion before placing it on the resident.

♥ 5. Make long, firm strokes along spine from buttocks to shoulders. Make circular strokes down on shoulders, upper arms and back to buttocks.

👩 Note that there are 2 different strokes to the back rub and don't miss the arms and shoulders!

♥ 6. Repeat for at least 3-5 minutes.

👩 Tester will have you verbalize the time frame and you need to know it exactly!

♥ 7. Gently pat off excess lotion with towel. Cover and position as resident requests.

👩 Patting off the excess lotion onto a towel has gotten missed...know this!

PROCEDURE #36: ORAL CARE - ALERT AND ORIENTED RESIDENT

2. Raise head of bed so resident is sitting up.

3. Put on gloves.

4. Drape towel under resident's chin.

The tester will ask "what would you do to protect your resident?".

5. Wet toothbrush and put on apply small amount of toothpaste.

This is typically how people brush their own teeth. Wet the toothbrush first just like you would for yourself.

6. First brush upper teeth and then lower teeth.

In this order or the tester will count this as a stop.

7. Hold emesis basin under resident's chin.

8. Ask resident to rinse mouth with water and spit into emesis basin.

9. If requested, give resident mouthwash diluted with half water.

Remember to bring mouthwash and cup with you to the bedside with supplies as students tend to forget this item.

10. Check teeth, mouth, tongue and lips for odor, cracking, sores, bleeding, discoloration and loose teeth. Report unusual findings to nurse.

You are checking 4 things MLTT. You are checking for 6 things OCSBDL. You need to remember this because you will always assess when providing any type of oral care for a resident.

11. Remove towel and wipe resident's mouth.

Since students are simulating this on the testing resident they forget to wipe the residents mouth. Just perform the RCP during the test as if it were real life!

12. Remove gloves.

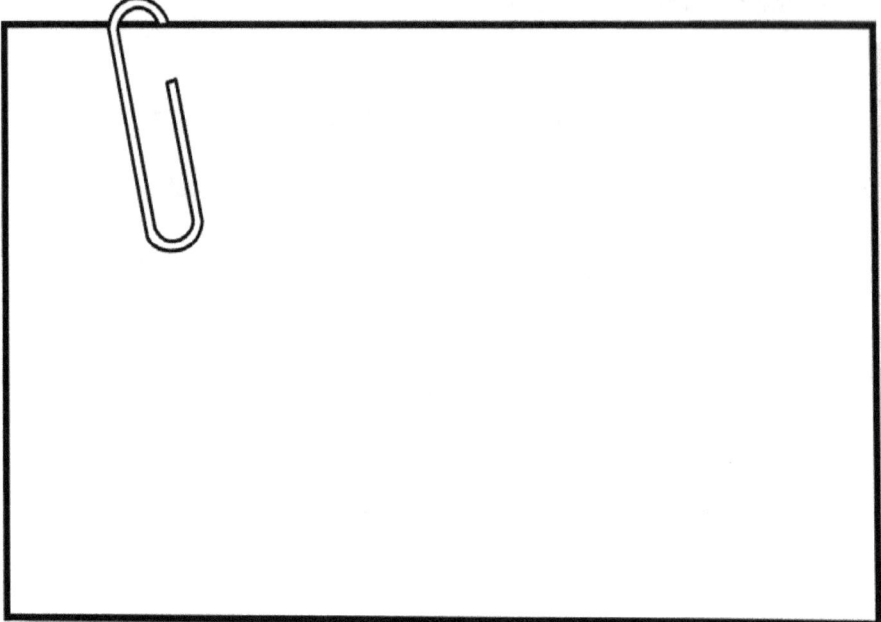

PROCEDURE #37: ORAL CARE FOR AN UNCONSCIOUS RESIDENT

2. Drape towel over pillow and a towel under resident's chin.

Bring 2 towels as part of your supplies!

Set supplies up on unaffected side.

3. Turn resident onto unaffected side.

Remember you will be turning the resident to the lateral position which will require you to put up the side rail prior to turning.

When you have turned the resident and have moved over to the unaffected side to start the procedure, make sure you put the side rail down and DO NOT LEAN OVER THE RAIL (safety caution stop).

4. Put on gloves.

5. Place an emesis basin under resident's chin.

6. Dip swab in cleaning solution of 1/2 mouthwash and 1/2 water and wipe teeth, gums, tongue and inside surfaces of mouth, changing swab frequently.

7. Rinse with clean swab dipped in water.

8. Check teeth, mouth, tongue and lips for odor, cracking, sores, bleeding, discoloration and loose teeth. Report unusual findings to nurse.

You are checking 4 things MLTT. You are checking for 6 things OCSBDL. You need to remember this because you always assess when providing any type of oral care for a resident.

9. Cover lips with thin layer of lip moisturizer.

You moisturize resident lips when providing denture care and when the resident is unconscious.

10. Remove gloves.

PROCEDURE #38: DENTURE CARE

2. Raise head of bed so resident is sitting up.

3. Put on gloves.

4. Drape towel under resident's chin.

5. Remind resident that you are going to remove their dentures. Remove Upper dentures by placing your index finger at the ridge on top of the right upper denture and gently moving them up and down to release suction. Turn lower denture slightly to lift out of mouth.

Students have missed removing dentures during the test. Make sure you understand step 5 EXACTLY and how to remove both top and bottom dentures.

6. Put dentures in denture cup marked with resident's name and take to sink.

7. Line sink with towel and fill halfway with water.

Dentures are expensive and very important to the residents. Putting a towel in the sink will help to make sure the dentures are safe.

8. Apply denture cleaner to toothbrush

9. Hold dentures over sink and brush all surfaces.

The reason for holding them over the sink with a towel in place is to prevent breakage...the tester may ask you this.

10. Rinse dentures under warm water, place in a clean cup and fill with cool water.

11. Clean resident's mouth with swab if necessary. Help resident rinse mouth with water or mouthwash diluted with half water, if requested.

12. Check teeth, mouth, tongue and lips for odor, cracking, sores, bleeding, discoloration and loose teeth. Report unusual findings

to nurse.

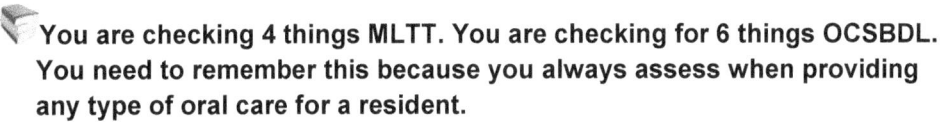You are checking 4 things MLTT. You are checking for 6 things OCSBDL. You need to remember this because you always assess when providing any type of oral care for a resident.

13. Help resident place dentures in mouth, if requested. Moisturize the lips.

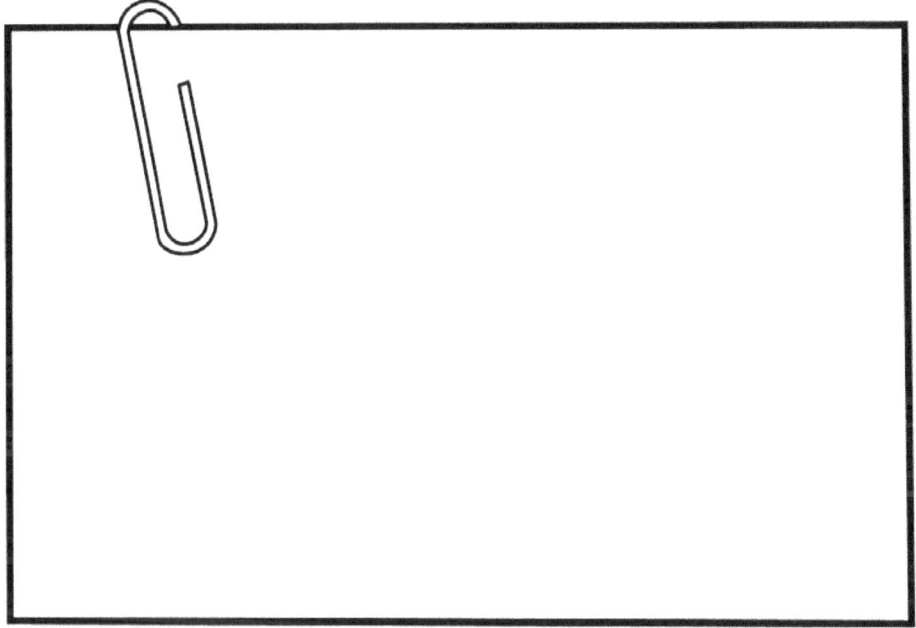You moisturize resident lips when providing denture care and when the resident is unconscious.

14. Remove gloves.

PROCEDURE #39: ELECTRIC RAZOR

2. Raise head of bed so resident is sitting up.

3. Do not use electric razor near any water source, when oxygen is in use or if resident has pacemaker.

Some students will bring the shaving cream with them as part of supplies to the bedside. Read the first ingredient in shaving cream...WATER!

This is another example of something that is in my Quizlet. You need to remember when to NOT use an electric razor.

4. Drape towel under resident's chin.

This is used in a handful of RCPs as well. Just be sure when you provide care for a resident you also place a towel under their chin for any water that may drip.

5. Put on gloves.

6. Apply pre-shave lotion as resident requests.

7. Hold skin taut and shave resident's face and neck according to manufacturer's guidelines.

Know the difference between how you hold the skin with electric versus safety razor as students WILL get this confused.

8. Check for any breaks in the skin. Apply after-shave lotion as resident requests.

9. Remove towel from resident.

10. Remove gloves.

PROCEDURE #40: SAFETY RAZOR

2. Raise head of bed so resident is sitting up.

On review day students tend to question whether to sit the resident up or not. Of course! Why would you make this procedure harder on yourself?

3. Fill bath basin halfway with warm water.

In all procedures that requires a basin it is ALWAYS filled halfway!

4. Drape towel under resident's chin.

The tester will state "what are you going to do to protect your resident?".

5. Put on gloves.

6. Moisten beard with washcloth and spread shaving cream over area.

Make sure you moisten with a washcloth FIRST before applying shaving cream. Bringing a washcloth with you to the bedside as part of your supplies. It will help to remind you of this step during the test.

7. Hold skin taut and shave beard in downward strokes on face and upward strokes on neck.

Know the difference between how you hold the skin with electric versus safety razor as students WILL get this confused.

8. Rinse resident's face and neck with washcloth.

Remember you are working with older people. You have to be careful because they have fragile skin and pulling it taut will help protect your resident from any cuts or sores. As for razor strokes, you will be going

with the hair growth...down on the face and up on the neck.

9. Pat dry with towel.

10. Apply after-shave lotion, as requested.

11. Remove towel.

12. Remove gloves.

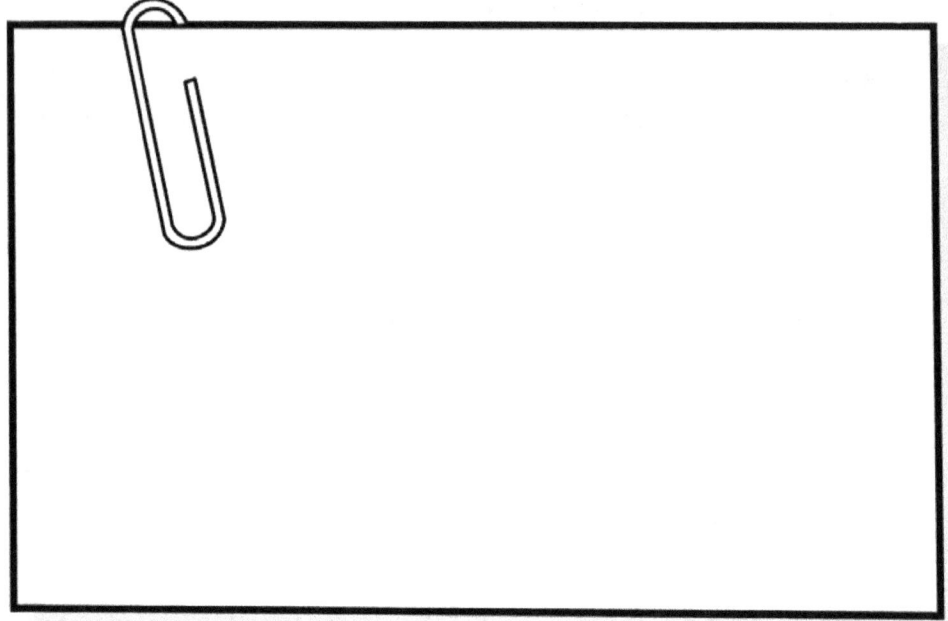

PROCEDURE #41: COMB/BRUSH HAIR

2. Raise head of bed so resident is sitting up.

3. **Drape towel over pillow.**

 This will catch the excess hair that falls.

4. Remove resident's glasses and any hairpins or clips.

5. Remove tangles by dividing hair into small sections and gently combing out from the ends of hair to scalp.

Students have forgotten this step. Make sure you repeat it from memorization during the test even if your testing resident has short hair. The entire step needs to be verbalized for the test.

6. Use hair products, as resident requests.

7. Style hair as resident requests.

8. Offer mirror.

 You can think of this as part of resident rights. They still care about how they look as much as you might.

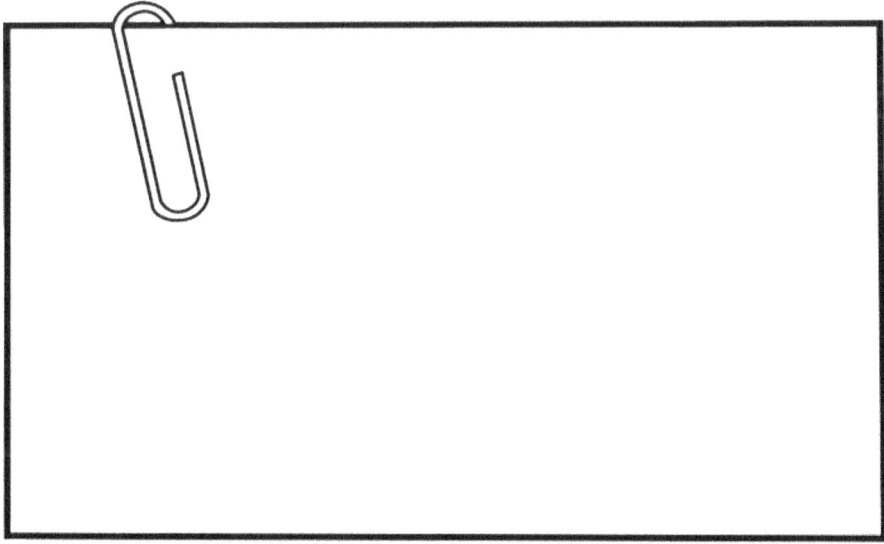

PROCEDURE #42: FINGERNAIL CARE

2. **Check fingers and nails for color, swelling, cuts or splits. Check hands for extreme heat or cold. Report any unusual findings to nurse before continuing procedure.**

Students will forget this important first step. Remember ASSESSING and reporting unusual findings to the nurse is ALWAYS a priority and the first step with many of the procedures.

3. Raise head of bed so resident is sitting up.

4. **Fill bath basin halfway** with warm water and have resident check water temperature for comfort.

In all procedures that a require a basin it is ALWAYS filled halfway!

5. Soak resident's hands and pat dry.

6. Put on gloves.

7. **Clean under nails with orange stick.**

Don't forget this step. Think about when you get your nails done at a salon. They clean under your nails as well.

8. Clip fingernails straight across, then file in a curve.

9. Remove gloves.

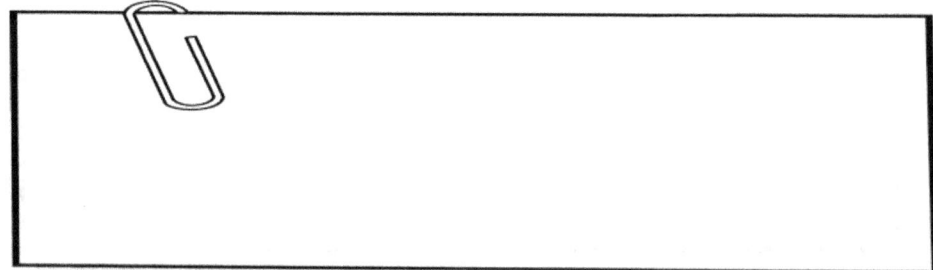

PROCEDURE #44: CHANGING RESIDENT'S GOWN

2. Untie soiled gown.

3. Raise top sheet over resident's chest.

📎 **Remember you need to provide privacy.**

♥ **4.** Remove resident's arms from gown, **unaffected arm first.**

♥ **5. Roll soiled gown from neck down and remove from beneath top sheet.** Place soiled gown in dirty linen bag.

♥ **6.** Slide resident's arms into clean gown, **affected arm first.**

👩 **During this step, the gown is on top of the sheets to provide privacy until both arms are in and gown is tied.**

👩 **GOLDEN RULE: Off first on the UNAFFECTED arm; On first on the AFFECTED arm!**

7. Tie gown.

8. Remove top sheet from beneath clean gown and cover resident.

👩 **During this step, the gown is on top of the sheets to provide privacy until the gown is tied. Then you would pull the sheet down and cover the resident. Remember privacy is ALWAYS a priority!**

PROCEDURE #45: DRESSING A DEPENDENT RESIDENT

2. Assist resident to choose clothing.

Remember it is a resident's right to choose their clothing. Don't forget to bring 2 choices of outfits for the resident to choose from during the test.

3. Move resident onto back.

4. Provide privacy.

Always use a bath blanket or sheet for this.

5. Guide feet through leg openings of underwear and pants, **affected leg first. Pull garments up legs to buttocks.**

6. Slide arm into shirt sleeve, **affected side first.**

7. Turn resident onto unaffected side. **Pull lower garments over buttocks and hip.** Tuck shirt under resident.

8. Turn resident onto affected side. **Pull lower garments over buttocks and hip** and straighten shirt.

Missed steps for this procedure include pulling up garments and tucking as much as possible prior to turning the resident. Your goal is to move the resident the least amount of times as possible.

9. Turn resident onto back and slide arm into shirt sleeve, align and fasten garments.

PROCEDURE #47: BEDSIDE COMMODE

2. Assist resident to put on non-skid socks/ footwear.

♥ 3. Place commode next to bed on resident's **unaffected side.**

Remember to always place a sitting device on the UNAFFECTED/ STRONG side.

Students have failed this procedure with 1-2" left between the bed and wheelchair. MAKE SURE it is braced firmly with NO SPACE between the chair and bed.

♥ 4. Assist resident to **transfer to commode by transferring the safest way** the resident is able.

What the tester is looking for here is using a gait belt. Most likely the scenario you will be given is with an affected side so for SAFETY you WILL use a gait belt to transfer to the bedside commode.

5. Give resident call light and toilet tissue if resident has been identified as safe to be provided privacy and not attended by staff.

6. Put on gloves.

7. Assist resident to wipe from front to back.

8. Wash hands and change gloves

When you're testing you don't actually have to change your gloves. You may just verbalize this to the tester.

9. Assist resident to bed or chair.

♥ 10. Remove and **cover pan** and take to bathroom.

Bring paper towel with you when you are gathering your supplies to cover pan.

♥ 11. Prior to disposal, observe urine and/or feces for color, odor, amount and characteristics and report unusual findings to nurse.

REMEMBER: COCA = Color, Odor, Consistency, Amount

Again, this is something that you do whenever you dispose of a residents output. The tester will ask you about this.

12. Dispose of urine and/or feces, sanitize pan and return pan according to facility policy.

13. Remove gloves. Wash hands

♥ 14. Assist resident to wash hands.

This get missed a lot. The tester may prompt "what do you need to do for infection control for your resident?".

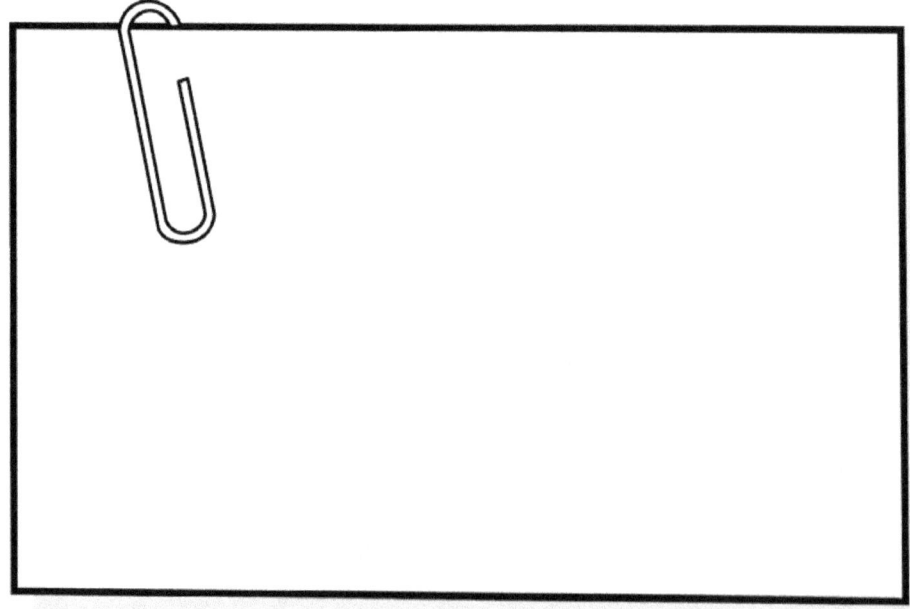

PROCEDURE #48: BEDPAN/FRACTURE PAN

2. Lower head of bed.

3. Put on gloves.

At this point, put up side rail on the opposite side you are going to turn the resident toward. **Never lean over the side rail once it is up (safety caution stop).**

4. Turn resident away from you.

5. Place bedpan or fracture pan under buttocks according to manufacturer directions.

The tester will allow you to choose either a fracture or regular bedpan.

REMEMBER: The large opening goes toward the head of the bed and small opening toward the foot.

6. Gently roll resident back onto pan and check for correct placement.

7. Cover resident with sheet/blanket.

PRIORITY: Resident privacy.

8. Raise head of bed to comfortable position for resident.

Seriously let's think this one through...what position would be easier for the resident to use the bedpan? If you do not put the head of the bed up the tester will prompt "is there a more comfortable position for the resident?".

9. Give resident call light and toilet paper.

10. Leave resident and return when called.

11. Lower head of bed.

Make sure you do this as it not only makes it harder for you, but very difficult to remove a bedpan with the head up.

12. Press bedpan flat on bed and turn resident.

Don't think you will get away with just pulling out the bedpan during the test! The tester WILL be looking closely for this step and you holding down the bedpan so it does not flip and spill when turning the resident to remove it.

13. Wipe resident from front to back. Wash hands and change gloves.

The tester will ask you "is there a certain way you would clean the resident?"

14. Provide perineal care, if necessary.

15. Cover bedpan and take to bathroom.

Bring paper towel with you when gathering your supplies!

16. Check urine and/or feces for color, odor, amount and characteristics and report unusual findings to nurse.

REMEMBER: COCA = Color, Odor, Characteristics, Amount

You always check for this when providing care for residents and assessing their output. It is important to note because the tester wants to know what you are assessing before disposing of this output.

17. Dispose of urine and/or feces, sanitize pan and return pan according to facility policies.

18. Remove gloves. Wash hands

19. Assist resident to wash hands.

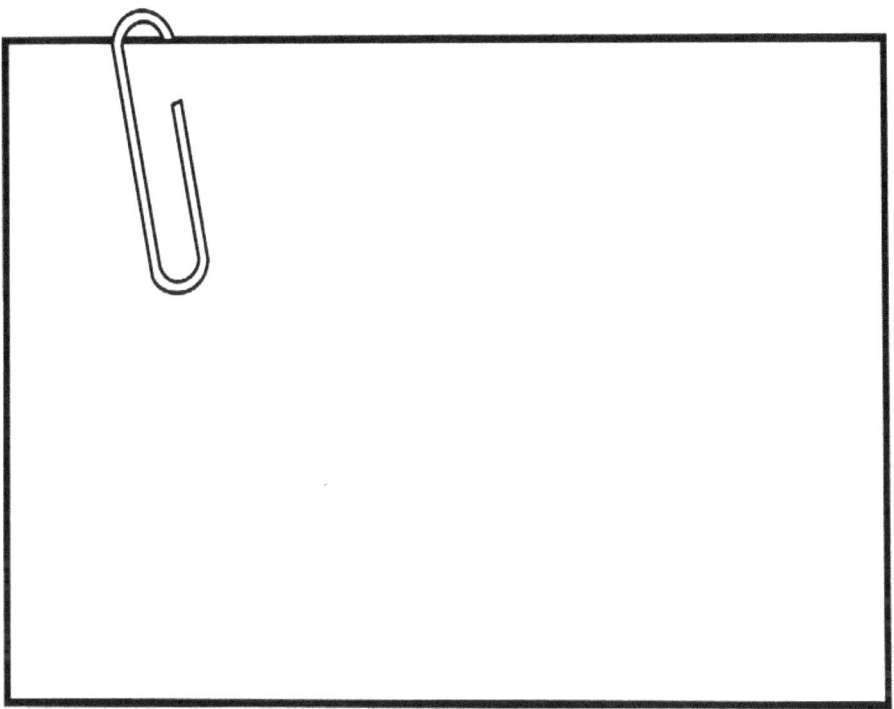
Many students get excited thinking the procedure is over… DON'T FORGET YOUR RESIDENT! The tester may prompt "is there something you should do for your resident for infection control?".

PROCEDURE #49: URINAL

2. Raise head of bed to sitting position.

Remember this is a more natural position for the resident to eliminate.

3. Put on gloves.

4. Offer urinal to resident or place urinal between his legs and insert penis into opening.

5. Cover resident.

6. Give resident call light and toilet paper.

7. Leave resident and return when called.

8. Remove and cover urinal.

Bring paper towel with you when you gather your supplies if the urinal does not have a cap attached.

9. Take urinal to bathroom, check urine for color, odor, amount and characteristics and report unusual findings to nurse.

REMEMBER: COCA = Color, Odor, Characteristics, Amount

You always check for this when providing care for residents and their output. It is important to note because the tester wants to know what you are assessing before disposing of this output.

10. Dispose of urine, rinse urinal, sanitize and return urinal according to facility policies.

11. Remove gloves. Wash hands

12. Assist resident to wash hands.

Many students get excited thinking the procedure is over…

DON'T FORGET YOUR RESIDENT! The tester may prompt "is there something you should do for your resident for infection control?"

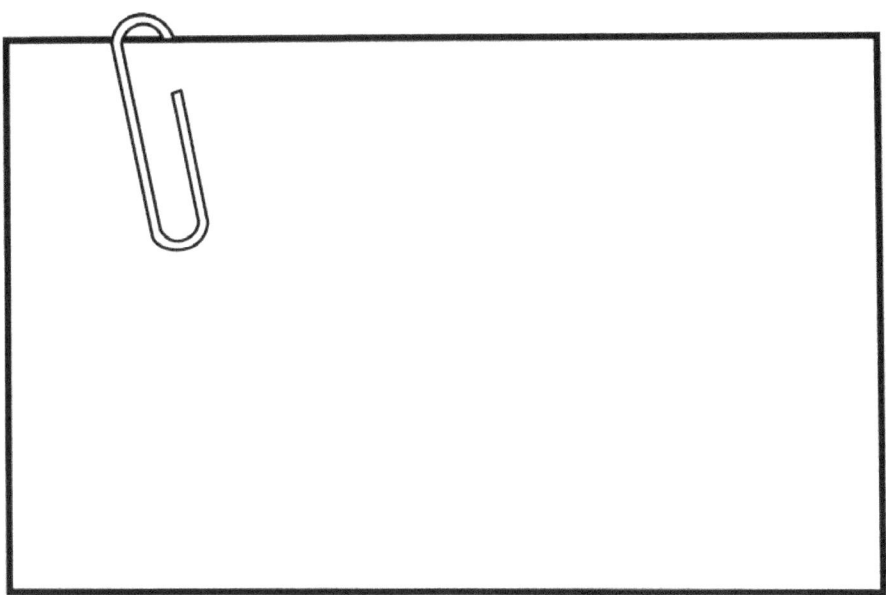

PROCEDURE #50: EMPTY URINARY DRAINAGE BAG

2. Put on gloves.

3. Place paper towel on floor beneath bag and place graduated cylinder on paper towel.

Remember to bring paper towel with you when gathering supplies.

4. Detach spout (if bag has one) and point the drainage tube into center of graduated cylinder without letting tube touch sides.

5. Unclamp spout and drain urine.

6. Clamp spout.

7. Replace spout in holder.

8. Check urine for color, odor, amount and characteristics and report unusual findings to nurse.

REMEMBER: COCA = Color, Odor, Characteristics, Amount

You always check for this when providing care for residents and their output. It is important to note because the tester wants to know what you are assessing before disposing of this output.

9. Measure and accurately record amount of urine.

Know how your testing site wants you to record I/O (cc or mm). Be ready to chart the amount on your procedure test sheet. The tester will ask you "show me where 300cc (or 300mm) is located on the graduated cylinder?". If you are correct, then the tester will have you document 300cc (or 300mm) in the output section of your procedure sheet.

10. Dispose of urine, rinse, sanitize and return graduated cylinder according to facility policies.

According to facility policies is a key note here. Again, do not say "that isn't how we do it at my facility" because the tester is not worried about your facility, they want to know the skills according to the RCP.

11. Remove gloves.

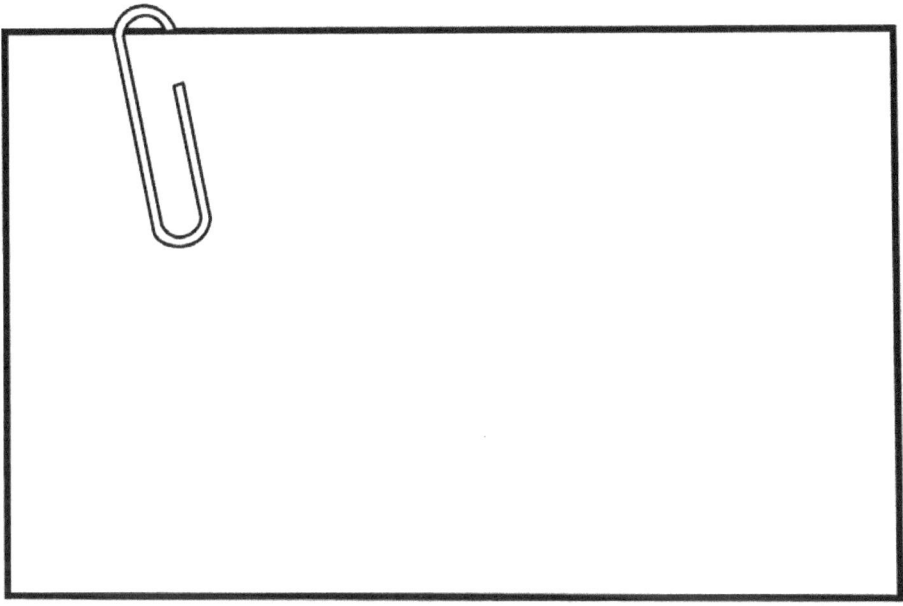

PROCEDURE #54: UNOCCUPIED BED

2. Collect clean linen in order of use.

3. Carry linen away from your uniform

4. Place linen on clean surface (bedside stand, overbed table or back of chair).

5. Place bed in flat position.

♥**6.** Loosen soiled linen. **Roll linen from head to foot of bed** and place in barrel at door or room or in bag and place at foot of bed or chair.

7. Fanfold bottom sheet to center of bed and fit corners.

This step is sometimes hard for students due to the popularity of fitted sheets with elastic all the way around. I have found tucking into the middle at the top and then working your way down will make this easier...however sometimes it feels like you are working with a Slinky!

When you do get it to "grab" the bed and then fanfold the top sheet (step 8) on top this seems to hold it in place at that point.

Bottom line...practice makes perfect!

8. Fanfold top sheet to center of bed.

9. Fanfold blanket over top sheet.

♥**10.** Tuck top linen under foot of mattress and **miter corner.**

Miter that corner well so the blanket and sheet are not touching the floor (infection control stop).

11. Move to other side of bed.

♥**12.** Fit corners of bottom sheet, unfold top linen, tuck it under foot of mattress, and **miter corner.**

13. Fold top of sheet over blanket to make cuff.

♥ **14. With one hand, grasp the clean pillow case at the closed end, turning it inside out over your arm.**

♥ **15. Using the same hand that has the pillowcase over it, grasp one narrow edge of the pillow and pull the pillowcase over it with your free hand.**

♥ **16. Place the pillow at head of bed with open edge away from the door.**

For steps 13, 14 and 15 practice, practice, practice as this is always stumbled over during the test. You are wanting to not touch the outside of the pillowcase....this is your goal!

ALWAYS open edge away from the door...many stops on this one!

17. For open bed: make toe pleat and fanfold top linen to foot of bed with top edge closest to center of bed.

An OPEN BED allows the resident to pull up the covers in 1 motion without any strain or with one easy movement. This usually refers to a bed that is occupied.

18. For closed bed: pull bedspread over pillow and tuck bedspread under lower edge of pillow. Make toe pleat.

A CLOSED BED usually refers to a bed that is ready for a new admission.

19. Removed soiled linens.

IMPORTANT: Making both types of beds have been very difficult procedures for students. Bottom line....practice and memorize these steps!

PROCEDURE #55: OCCUPIED BED

2. Collect clean linen in order of use.

3. Carry linen away from your uniform

4. Place linen on clean surface (bedside stand, overbed table or back of chair).

5. Lower head of bed and adjust bed to a safe working level, usually waist high. Lock bed wheels.

6. Drape the resident

Utilizing the bath sheet is the easiest way to provide privacy.

During testing your resident will have clothes on, but always remember that you need to provide privacy. This can be done with a sheet or a bath blanket.

7. The caregiver will make the bed one side at a time. The caregiver will raise the side rail on far side of bed (if rail not in use, ensure there is a second caregiver on the opposite side of the bed to ensure that the resident does not roll over the side of bed). Assist resident to turn onto side moving away from you toward raised side rail (or second caregiver).

REMEMBER: Do not lean over the side rail you have just raised (safety caution stop).

8. Loosen bottom soiled linen on the side of bed on which you are working.

9. Roll bottom soiled linen toward resident and tuck it snugly against the resident's back.

10. Place clean bottom linen on unoccupied side of bed and roll remaining clean linen under resident in the center of the bed.

This step is sometimes hard for students due to the popularity of fitted sheets with elastic all the way around. Making an occupied bed is easier because you can tuck the top of the sheet under the residents head which

will hold it down while working your way down the bed.

♥ **11. Smooth bottom sheet out and ensure there are no wrinkles.** Roll all extra material toward resident and tuck it under the resident's body.

Wrinkles = bed sores. The tester will be looking so make sure you don't have any.

Making sure that there are no wrinkles is to prevent pressure ulcers.

♥ **12. Raise the side rail nearest you** (or remain in place if a second caregiver is being utilized) and assist the resident to turn onto clean bottom sheet. Move to opposite side of bed, as resident will now be facing away from you.

REMEMBER: DO NOT lean over the bed railing as this is a safety caution stop. Where students make this mistake is raising the side rail, then see a sheet or blanket that could be straightened after they have put it up and reach over get the stop!

♥ **13.** While resident is lying on side, **loosen soiled linen and roll linen from head to foot of bed,** avoiding contact with your skin or clothing.

Remember ALWAYS head to toe and out the side or you will have an infection control stop!

14. Place soiled linen in barrel or bag at foot of bed or in chair.

15. Pull clean bottom linen as was done on the opposite side.

♥ **16. Assist resident to roll onto back, keeping resident covered and comfortable.**

Again, with PRIVACY! Utilize your bath blanket here!

17. Unfold the top sheet placing it over the resident. Request the resident to hold the clean top sheet. While slipping the bath blanket or previous sheet out from underneath the clean sheet.

♥ **18.** Assist resident with blanket over the top sheet and tuck the bottom edges of the top sheet and blanket under the bottom of the mattress. **Miter the corners and loosen the top linens over the resident's feet.**

Miter those corners! If they fall on the floor you will have an infection control caution stop!

Don't forget to loosen the linens at the feet. I have seen this missed. It prevents foot drop!

If you do not understand this you can always look it up on YouTube. I relate mitering corners to making a sailboat with the end of the sheet and tucking the bottom part in.

♥ **19.** Remove pillow and remove the soiled pillow case by turning it inside out.

♥ **20.** With one hand, grasp the clean pillow case at the closed end, turning it inside out over your arm.

♥ **21.** Using the same hand that has the pillowcase over it, grasp one Narrow edge of the pillow and pull the pillowcase over it with your free hand

♥ **22.** Place the pillow under resident's head with open edge away from the door.

For steps 19, 20, 21 and 22 practice, practice, practice as this is always stumbled over during the test. You are wanting to not touch the outside of the pillowcase... this is your goal!

ALWAYS open edge away from the door...stops on this one!

23. Assist resident to comfortable position and return the bed to the appropriate position.

24. Removed soiled linens from room – carrying away from uniform.

IMPORTANT: Making both types of beds have been very difficult procedures for students. Bottom line... practice and memorize these steps!

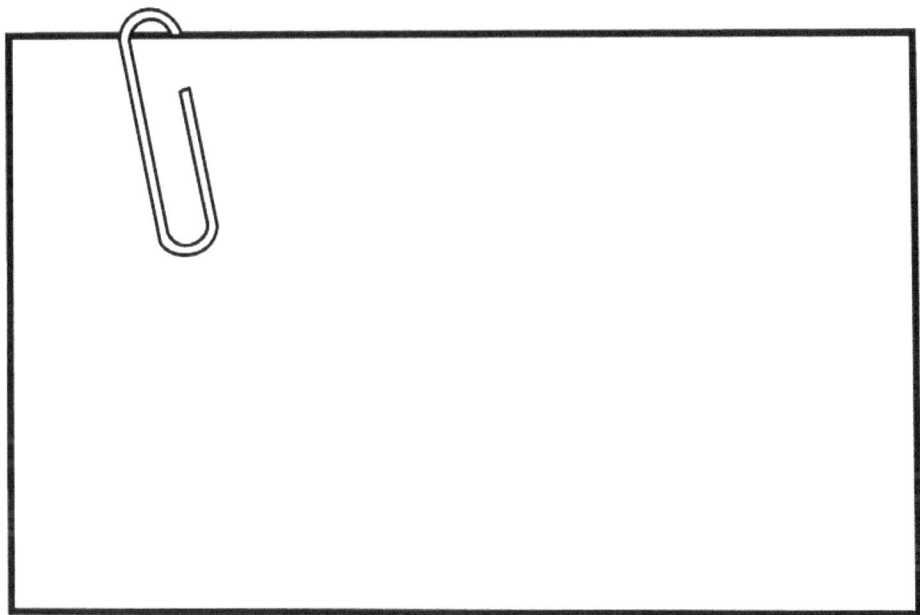

PROCEDURE #60: INSPECTING SKIN

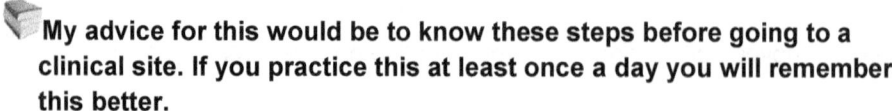 My advice for this would be to know these steps before going to a clinical site. If you practice this at least once a day you will remember this better.

2. Provide the resident privacy.

3. Check bony areas including ears, shoulder blades, elbows, coccyx, hips, knees, ankles and heels for redness and warmth.

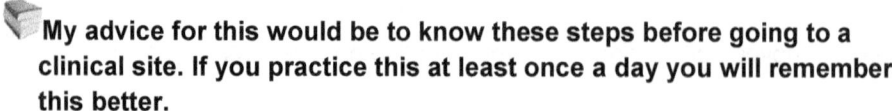 **You are checking 8 bony areas for redness and warmth.**

4. Check friction areas including under breasts and arms, between buttocks, groin, thighs, skin folds, contracted areas, and around any tubing for redness, irritation, moisture and odor.

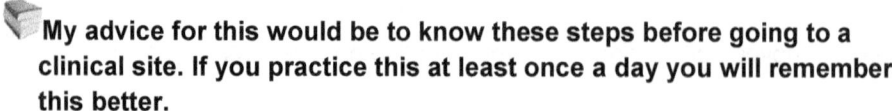 **You are checking 7 friction areas for redness, irritation, moisture and odor - RIMO.**

5. Undrape resident.

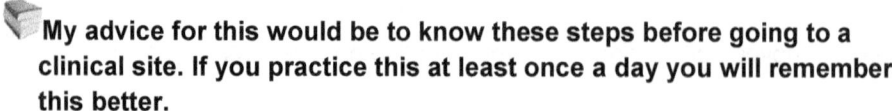 **Again, privacy is important.**

6. Report any unusual findings to the nurse immediately.

The tests that I have observed, the tester will have you verbalize the areas and steps of this procedure. Bottom line...memorize EXACTLY!

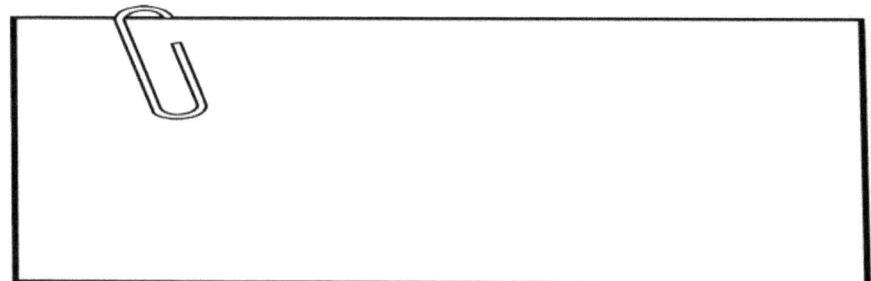

PROCEDURE #61: FLOAT HEELS

2. Lift resident's lower extremity.

3. Inspect the skin, especially the heels.

Even though it doesn't say it here, verbalizing to the tester that you would assess and report any abnormal findings to the nurse would be a **GOOD THING!**

4. **Place a full pillow under calves, leaving heels in the air and free from pressure.** (Do not use rolled pillows or blankets.)

I have seen students do this procedure perfectly EXCEPT the heels are on top of the pillow. The procedure is called FLOAT HEELS... the heels should be off the pillow and floating.

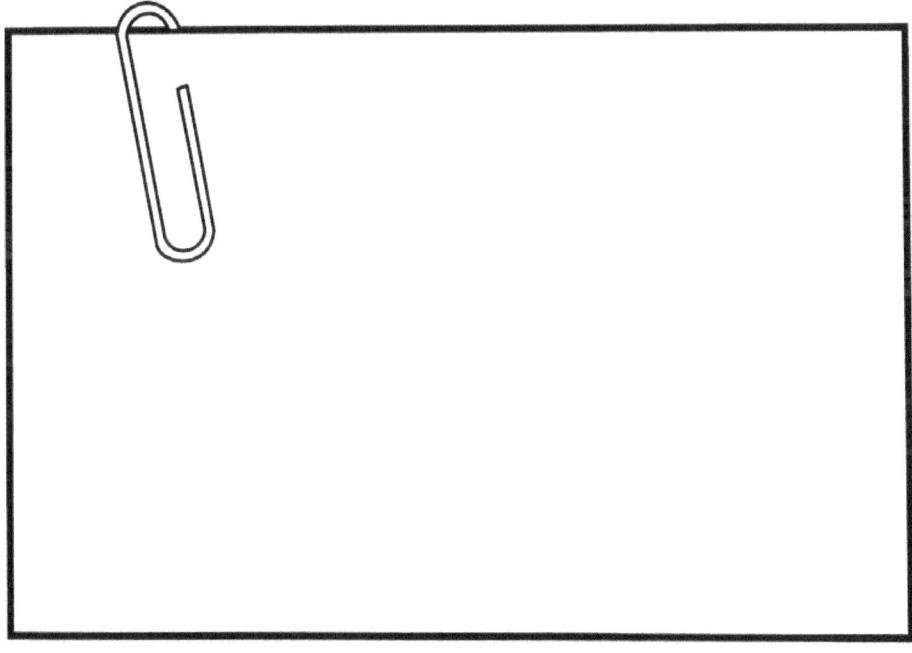

PROCEDURE #63: PASSIVE RANGE OF MOTION

2. Position resident in good body alignment.

♥ 3. Observe joints. If swelling, redness or warmth is present, or if resident complains of pain, notify nurse. Continue procedure only if instructed.

👩‍⚕️ Many students will start right into PROM. Remember you always assess first and report any abnormal findings.

📖 These are some of things I have on my Quizlet.

♥ 4. Support limb above and below joint.

👩‍⚕️ Students have been stopped due to not supporting joints correctly. If you think about it, you really can't do the exercise right if you don't support the limbs this way.

♥ 5. Begin range of motion at shoulders and include the shoulders, elbows, wrists, thumbs, fingers, hips, knees, ankles and toes.

6. Slowly move joint in all directions it normally moves.

📖 Don't overthink this. Just move them how you would feel comfortable moving your own joints.

♥ 7. Repeat movement at least five times.

8. Encourage resident to participate as much as possible.

9. Stop procedure at any sign of pain and report to nurse immediately.

👩‍⚕️ The tester will ask you "what would be a reason you would stop this procedure?". Know that PAIN is a cardinal sign of something going on with the resident. The procedure should be stopped immediately and notify the nurse.

The Authors:

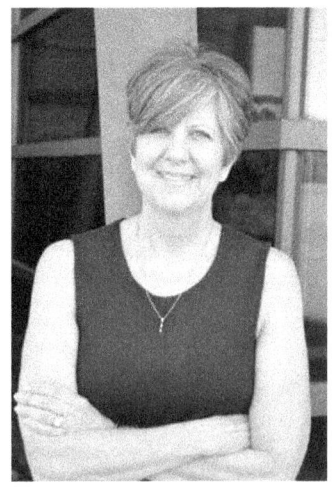

Juli Murphy RN, BSN
CNA Program Director
Premier Nursing Academy
Juli graduated from Indiana Wesleyan University in 2006 with a Bachelor of Science degree in Nursing. She started her nursing career in 1978 as a CNA then graduated from Fort Wayne Community School of Practical Nursing in 1980. She received her Associate of Science in Nursing from the University of St. Francis in 2002. She currently manages the CNA program for Premier Nursing Academy which includes supervision of instructors and students, ongoing programing and expansion to outlying cities. She is married to Richard and together they have 5 children, 9 grandchildren, 3 great grandchildren and a Giant Schnoodle named Charlie.

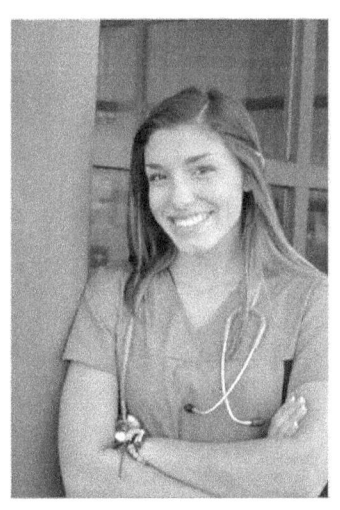

Katlyn Friend-Setser CNA
RCP Peer Reviewer/Peer-Peer Mentor
Premier Nursing Academy
Katlyn graduated from Leo High School in 2017. She is moving forward in healthcare working toward her Bachelor of Science degree in Nursing from Purdue University. She received a CNA license during her Senior year from Premier Nursing Academy and will continue that work until finishing her degree. She also instructs ongoing review classes for Premier helping mentor peers to pass the state exam. There are so many things she would like to accomplish and truly believes it will be a breeze

with her own mini fan club consisting of her mother, father, 2 younger brothers and 2 wonderful sets of grandparents.

www.ingramcontent.com/pod-product-compliance
Lightning Source LLC
Chambersburg PA
CBHW050237230526
45470CB00005B/1995